Difficult Cases in Primary Care: Women's Health

SAMAR RAZAQ

MBChB, MRCGP, DRCOG, DCH, DGM

General Practitioner
Buckinghamshire

Radcliffe Publishing
London • New York

Radcliffe Publishing Ltd
33–41 Dallington Street
London
EC1 V 0BB
United Kingdom

www.radcliffepublishing.com

#812184887

Every effort has been made to ensure that the information in this book is accurate. This does not diminish the requirement to exercise clinical judgement, and neither the publisher nor the author can accept any responsibility for its use in practice.

British Library Cataloguing in Publication Data

A catalogue record for this book is available from the British Library.

ISBN-13: 978 184619 511 2

Typeset by Beautiful Words, Auckland, New Zealand
Printed and bound by Cadmus Communications, USA

Contents

Preface

Men and women differ in their biological makeup, which results in a different set of conditions affecting the two sexes. Moreover, similar conditions may present differently in men and women. Pregnancy, lactation and the menstrual cycle are unique to women and bring challenges to the general practitioner in terms of diagnosis and management. Therefore, it is important to have a good grasp of difficult scenarios that may arise in the consultation room.

This book covers important topics concerning women's health through clinical scenarios, giving the reader the opportunity to observe how such conditions may present in real life and be managed. The following exam-style questions test the reader's knowledge of the topic before a detailed explanation of how the case may be managed is given. The scenarios are described to suit the various exams in which the candidate is provided with relevant information prior to seeing the patient. This provides practice for the objective structured clinical exams (OSCEs) that many medical students and specialty trainees have to take and also for the clinical skills assessment (CSA) for general practice trainees. Each scenario is supplemented with extended matching questions (EMQs), single best answer questions (SBAs) and multiple-choice questions (MCQs) that complement the clinical scenarios and give a broader overview of related clinical situations, providing valuable exam preparation for exam candidates.

Samar Razaq

June 2012

List of abbreviations

ACE	angiotensin-converting enzyme
AMAs	anti-mitochondrial antibodies
ARTs	assisted reproductive techniques
AV	aerobic vaginitis
BMD	bone mineral density
BMI	body mass index
BP	blood pressure
BV	bacterial vaginosis
CBT	cognitive behavioural therapy
CHD	coronary heart disease
CO	carbon monoxide
CNS	central nervous system
COCPs	combined oral contraceptive pills
CRS	congenital rubella syndrome
CSA	clinical skills assessment
CT	computed tomography
CTG	cardiotocography
CTPA	computed tomography pulmonary angiogram
DEET	*N,N*-Diethyl-*meta*-toluamide

DEXA	dual-energy X-ray absorptiometry
DVT	deep vein thrombosis
ECT	electroconvulsive therapy
ECV	external cephalic version
EMQs	extended matching questions
FBC	full blood count
FRAX	*FRAX® WHO Fracture Risk Assessment Tool*
FSD	female sexual dysfunction
FSH	follicle stimulating hormone
FVS	fetal varicella syndrome
GnRH	gonadotrophin-releasing hormone
GTD	gestational trophoblastic disease
GTN	gestational trophoblastic neoplasia
HBV	hepatitis B virus
hCG	human chorionic gonadotrophin
HCV	hepatitis C virus
HELLP	haemolysis, elevated liver enzymes and low platelet count
HG	hyperemesis gravidarum
HIV	human immunodeficiency virus
HNIG	human normal immunoglobulin
HRT	hormone replacement therapy
HPA	Health Protection Agency
HPV	human papillomavirus
HSV	herpes simplex virus
Ig	immunoglobulin
IUGR	intrauterine growth restriction
LARCs	long-acting reversible contraceptives
LDL	low-density lipoprotein
LFT	liver function test
LH	luteinising hormone
LLETZ	large loop excision of the transformation zone
LOS	laparoscopic ovarian surgery

LRs	likelihood ratios
MAOIs	monoamine oxidase inhibitors
MASI	Melasma Area and Severity Index
MCQs	multiple-choice questions
NSAIDs	non-steroidal anti-inflammatory drugs
NICE	National Institute for Health and Clinical Excellence
NRT	nicotine replacement therapy
OAB	overactive bladder
OSCEs	objective structured clinical exams
PBC	primary biliary cirrhosis
PCOS	polycystic ovarian syndrome
PCR	polymerase chain reaction
PMS	premenstrual syndrome
PND	postnatal depression
POP	progestogen-only pill
PTH	parathyroid hormone
RAADP	routine antenatal anti-D prophylaxis
RCT	randomised controlled trial
RhD	rhesus D
RMI	Risk of Malignancy Index
SBAs	single best answer questions
SCD	sickle cell disease
SFH	symphysis–fundal height
SHBG	sex hormone-binding globulin
SSPE	subacute sclerosing panencephalitis
SSRI	selective serotonin reuptake inhibitor
STI	sexually transmitted infection
TCAs	tricyclic antidepressants
TG	triglyceride
TSH	thyroid-stimulating hormone
USS	ultrasound scan
VQ	ventilation-perfusion lung scan

VTE   venous thromboembolism

VZIG   varicella zoster immunoglobulin

VZV   varicella zoster virus

UKMEC *UK Medical Eligibility Criteria for Contraceptive Use*

UPSI   unprotected sexual intercourse

Chickenpox in pregnancy

A nurse who you have worked with on the haematology ward confronts you in the corridor of the hospital. She is rather worried and seeks your advice. She is 20 weeks pregnant. She tells you that she has been looking after a patient with multiple mycloma on chemotherapy for the last week. As she attended to him this morning, she noticed that he had a rather blistery looking rash around his right eye. Since the patient was complaining of soreness, she applied some emollient to help with the discomfort. However, later during the ward round, the doctor had a look and confirmed herpes zoster ophthalmicus. She has never had chickenpox and her lack of immunity to chickenpox was confirmed on antenatal blood tests in her first trimester. She has no medical history of note.

What is the best advice you can give to this worried nurse?
a   Reassure and do nothing.
b   Reassure and advise her to seek help if a rash develops.
c   Organise a blood test for the nurse to check for varicella zoster virus (VZV) immunoglobulin (Ig) G antibody.
d   Admit as an emergency under the obstetric team.
e   Administer varicella zoster immunoglobulin (VZIG) as soon as possible.

f   Offer her varicella vaccine.

g   Reassure, as she is unlikely to develop chickenpox in pregnancy.

h   Advise termination due to severe complications of fetal varicella syndrome (FVS).

Answer: e

This scenario explores the circumstances around the exposure of pregnant women to VZV. Primary VZV infection, commonly known as chickenpox, is a common childhood disease. Exposure to it in pregnancy is also common but infection is not. It is an important condition in pregnancy due to the additional risks it poses to the pregnant mother and the fetus. Although it may be a mild self-limiting illness in children, it carries excess morbidity in adults. This is due to the greater risk of pneumonia, hepatitis, encephalitis and occasionally death. Chickenpox in pregnancy is associated with intrauterine growth restriction (IUGR), low birthweight and an increased risk of preterm delivery. In the fetus, there is an increased risk of developing FVS, an in utero syndrome of fetal congenital anomalies that may include skin scarring, defects of the eye, limb hypoplasia and neurological defects. Based on the dermatomal patterns of skin lesions in the infant, it is thought that FVS is caused by a reactivation of VZV in utero rather than by primary virus infection. This fact has a bearing on the timing of ultrasound for the prenatal diagnosis of FVS. Fetal infection can be determined by polymerase chain reaction (PCR) of amniotic fluid for VZV DNA. Although this has an excellent negative predictive value, positive predictive value has been reported to be poor. Therefore, diagnosis of FVS relies on a detailed ultrasound examination in which the deformities typical of the syndrome are sought. Since time must be allowed for reactivation of the virus and for these typical deformities to develop, a scan should be performed at least 5 weeks after the development of the maternal rash. Serial ultrasound scans (USSs) are likely to be required. This will be an anxious time for the mother and appropriate support and reassurance should be offered. The mother should be advised that there is an approximately 1 in 40 chance of the fetus developing FVS when primary VZV infection occurs in the first two trimesters of pregnancy. However, approximately one in three infants who develop FVS will die in the first few months of life. All cases of FVS have been reported when maternal infection occurs before 28 weeks, though it is particularly rare after 20 weeks.

Before discussing this particular case, it is worthwhile considering the alternative scenarios that may present in the same context.

1 Pregnant patient, with known immunity, exposed to VZV.

2 Pregnant patient, with doubtful immunity, exposed to VZV.

3 Pregnant patient, with known lack of immunity, exposed to VZV.

4 Patient with doubtful, or lack of, immunity, presenting for pre-conceptual advice.

5 Pregnant patient with chickenpox.

The first scenario is the most common situation that presents in primary care, as over 90% of the population of childbearing age in the UK is positive for varicella zoster IgG antibody (immunity amongst individuals from tropical climates is much lower). If there is a history suggestive of chickenpox, there is a 97%–99% chance of the patient having serum varicella antibodies. Therefore, it would be reasonable to consider such patients immune and offer reassurance. If, however, immunity is doubtful, as in the second scenario, then a blood test should be offered for confirmation of VZV immunity. This would usually be the case if the patient is unsure whether they had chickenpox in childhood. On blood testing, if immunity is confirmed, she has nothing to worry about. If, however, she is not immune, as in the third scenario, she will require VZIG. VZIG is a human-specific Ig (i.e. made from plasma containing high levels of VZV antibody titres) obtained from non-UK donors. It confers temporary immunity against the virus and is effective for 3 weeks. In this case, the nurse is not immune and she has had a high-risk exposure. Immunocompromised patients with exposed lesions, such as those in shingles of the ophthalmic nerve, present the highest risk of viral shedding; hence, the highest risk of transmitting the virus. Unexposed lesions, such as shingles of the thoracolumbar region, have a low risk of transmission. In this case, the patient should receive VZIG as soon as possible. VZIG is at its most effective when given within 72 hours of exposure. It should certainly be offered if the patient presents within 96 hours of exposure. Beyond this time, its effectiveness has not been evaluated, but some recommend administering it up to 10 days post-exposure.

The fourth scenario explores the scope of primary prevention in women seeking advice prior to becoming pregnant. A blood test should be offered to such women to check for VZV immunity. If the patient is not immune, vaccination against VZV should be offered. The varicella vaccine is a live attenuated virus. Although not part of the routine immunisation schedule in the UK, two varicella vaccines are licensed in the UK: Varivax® and Varilrix®. After vaccination, she should be advised to avoid pregnancy for 3 months and to avoid contact with other susceptible pregnant women should she develop a rash after the vaccination. Even though the vaccine is not offered in pregnancy, there is a register of cases in which it has been given to pregnant women accidentally. In such cases of inadvertent administration, there have been no reports of FVS and there does not appear to be an increase of fetal abnormalities above the baseline risk. It is worth noting that screening for VZV immunity is not part of routine antenatal care in the UK, despite a recent study demonstrating its cost-effectiveness in those with a negative history for chickenpox. Since women from tropical and subtropical areas are more likely to be non-immune to VZV, it is worth checking their immunity prenatally.

The final scenario is potentially serious due to the increased mortality and morbidity associated with varicella infection in pregnancy. Once clinical disease develops, VZIG is no longer effective. In this scenario, antiviral therapy should be used. Acyclovir and valacyclovir seem to be safe in pregnancy and are used at doses of 800 mg five times per day and 1 g three times per day for 7 days, respectively. If varicella pneumonia develops, the pregnant woman should be hospitalised; once there, antiviral treatment is usually administered intravenously.

Examination practice: infections in pregnancy

Options for questions 1–3:

a   reassure that risk of harm to fetus is very low and she should seek help if unwell

b   reassure and advise to seek help if a rash develops

c   refer urgently to an obstetrician

d   refer as an emergency to an obstetrician

e   refer urgently to termination of pregnancy services

f   review patient in 48 hours

g   perform serological tests

h   none of the above.

Instructions: The following questions refer to women contracting infections during pregnancy. Choose the most suitable management plan from options a–h. Each option may be used once, more than once or not at all.

1   A 38-year-old nursery worker presents to your surgery. She is 38 weeks pregnant. She has developed a localised rash on her back that is typical of shingles. She had chickenpox as a child.

2   A 22-year-old woman comes to you with a rash. She is 9 weeks pregnant and is worried about rubella as she has been in contact with a child with possible rubella infection.

3   A woman who is 36 weeks pregnant, with known non-immunity to rubella, presents with recent exposure to this virus.

4   Mark the following statements as either true or false.

   a   Chickenpox in pregnancy is complicated by maternal pneumonia in about 10%–20% of cases.

   b   The risk of maternal varicella pneumonia increases with increasing gestational age.

   c   The purpose of giving VZIG to a pregnant woman is to prevent FVS.

   d   Breastfeeding is contraindicated after VZV vaccination due to high levels of VZV DNA in breast milk.

   e   Survivors of FVS may develop long-term learning difficulties.

5 Indicate which of the following statements are true regarding measles in pregnancy.

    a Measles in pregnancy is rare due to the introduction of widespread immunisation.

    b Measles in the pregnant mother is strongly associated with a variety of congenital defects in the fetus.

    c Measles appears to be a mild illness in pregnancy with little or no increase in complications to the mother and fetus.

    d Measles late in pregnancy, leading to infection in the infant, may be associated with the risk of developing subacute sclerosing panencephalitis (SSPE).

    e National UK guidelines state that susceptible pregnant women should be given human normal immunoglobulin (HNIG) within 24 hours of exposure to measles.

References

Dontigny L, Arsenault M, Martel M. SOGC clinical practice guidelines: rubella in pregnancy. *J Obstet Gynaecol Can.* 2008; **30**(2): 152–8.

Gardella C, Brown ZA. Managing varicella zoster infection in pregnancy. *Cleve Clin J Med.* 2007; **74**(4): 290–6.

Lamont RF, Sobel JD, Carrington D, *et al.* Varicella-zoster (chickenpox) infection in pregnancy. *BJOG.* 2011; **118**(10): 1155–62.

Manikkavasagan G, Ramsay M. The rationale for use of measles post-exposure prophylaxis in pregnant women: a review. *J Obstet Gynaecol.* 2009; **29**(7): 572–5.

Royal College of Obstetricians and Gynaecologists (RCOG). *Chickenpox in Pregnancy.* Green-top Guideline No. 13. London: Guidelines and Audit Committee of the RCOG; September 2007. Available at: www.rcog.org. uk/files/rcog-corp/uploaded-files/GT13ChickenpoxinPregnancy2007.pdf (accessed 3 March 2012).

Depression in pregnancy

A 26-year-old woman presents to your clinic to inform you that she is 8 weeks pregnant. As you bring her records up on the computer, you immediately notice that she suffered from severe postnatal depression (PND) after the birth of her first child 3 years ago. This required admission on the mother and baby unit for 6 weeks. You question her further and she tells you that she felt low right through her first pregnancy but did not have the courage to discuss things with anyone. After the delivery, 'things got on top of her' and she 'just had a breakdown'. She then reveals that she has been feeling very similar since finding out she is pregnant and is wondering if there is any medication she could take to prevent a reoccurrence of the situation of her first pregnancy.

Which of the following statements are true?
a   Treatment of depression is multifaceted and multidisciplinary and medications can be a crucial part.
b   Monoamine oxidase inhibitors (MAOIs) are considered the first-line in the pharmaceutical management of depression.
c   Exposure to mirtazapine in the first trimester is an indicator for termination of pregnancy.

d   Neonatal adaptation syndrome, causing abnormal central nervous system (CNS), motor and respiratory signs, is associated with selective serotonin reuptake inhibitor (SSRI) use in pregnancy.

e   There is a possibility that SSRIs may increase the risk of fetal cardiac anomalies in first trimester exposure.

Answer: a, d and e

Depression may be encountered in up to one in five women in pregnancy. The patient in this case exhibits the strongest risk factor for developing depression in pregnancy – that is, a history of depression. Depression in pregnancy is more common in young single mothers with more than three children and an inadequate social support network. Depression in pregnancy not only affects the mother, it also has an adverse effect on the developing fetus and can impact on her relationship with her partner and on the care of any other children. The probability of recovery diminishes the longer the patient suffers from depression. It is vital, therefore, particularly in the context of pregnancy, to identify depression early and develop a management strategy.

Management of depression in a pregnant woman will share many features of that in her non-pregnant counterpart. Regular exercise (as recommended in a later case) should be advised. Psychotherapies such as CBT, though not extensively studied in pregnancy, should be offered when available. Data for alternative therapies for depression in pregnancy, such as St John's wort and acupuncture, are lacking. Although acupuncture has been used for other conditions in pregnancy with varying success, St John's wort should not be recommended in pregnancy due to the lack of data regarding how it may affect the pregnancy. When deciding whether to treat depression with pharmacotherapy, four risks need to be considered:

1   the risk of untreated depression to the mother
2   the risk of untreated depression to the fetus and infant
3   the risk of adverse effects of medication on the mother
4   the risk of adverse effects of medication on the fetus and infant.

As with all treatments, the physician should evaluate the benefits and risks of the treatment with respect to the individual patient. In the pregnant mother, depression affects the ability to perform routine daily tasks. She is more likely to turn to smoking, alcohol and illegal drugs, increasing the risk of harm to herself and to the fetus. At the extreme end of the spectrum, it may result in suicide. There is evidence to suggest that depression in pregnancy may impair important developmental aspects in the unborn child, including neurocognitive and socioemotional development. Untreated in the post-partum period, it will also impact the mother–child attachment, which may interfere with the child's psychological, educational and social development. These risks should be weighed against the potential risks of available drugs. It should be noted that data from randomised controlled trials (RCTs) for antidepressants are not available. A definite answer regarding the safety of drugs is unlikely, as the various prospective and retrospective studies, meta-analyses and population-based studies often have conflicting data. However, knowledge of the scale of risk and comparatively safer options is vital to help the patient and physician make an informed and appropriate decision.

Tricyclic antidepressants (TCAs) are generally used as first-line treatment in pregnancy due to experience of use and cumulative safety data. Amongst the TCAs, amitriptyline, nortriptyline, imipramine and desipramine may be considered the safest due to the greatest amount of accumulated safety data. They are not associated with an increased incidence of congenital anomalies above the background risk of 2%–4%. There is some suggestion of an asso-ciation between clomipramine and cardiac malformations, thus is therefore best avoided, especially as there are safer alternatives available in this group. However, TCAs must be avoided in mothers with suicidal tendencies due to their deleterious effects on both mother and child in the case of overdose. Another problem with TCAs is the greater incidence of anti-muscarinic side effects, which may be quite troublesome. TCAs have also been linked with an increased risk of delivery prior to 37 weeks. TCAs are excreted in breast milk. Non-sedating TCAs with a shorter half-life, such as imipramine and nortriptyline, are preferable as long as the child is born at term and healthy. Any risk to the child may be further minimised by using a once-daily dosing regimen (e.g. imipramine 75–150 mg taken once at night). The mother may alternate between breast and bottle-feeding to reduce drug levels in the infant. One should still be on the lookout for signs of sedation and irritability in the child. Specialist advice should be sought if breastfeeding in preterm unhealthy children is being considered. If the mother is very keen, one option could be to encourage expressing, to maintain milk production, but to start active breastfeeding once the child has grown and is in good health. Under these circumstances, advice would be given on a case-by-case basis.

It is very common to encounter women of childbearing age on SSRIs due to the frequency with which they are prescribed in this age group. Following exposure in the first trimester, there is a possibility that SSRIs double the risk of cardiac malformations, primarily septal defects, from 1% to 2%. Data from various studies are conflicting, but fluoxetine and paroxetine are the two SSRIs particularly implicated in this. Citalopram and sertraline appear to have a more favourable safety profile in pregnancy. However, individual studies have also implicated the latter two in this apparent increase in cardiac malformations, suggesting a possible drug class effect. The apparent contradiction in various studies is probably due to a host of confounding factors. For example, one study found infants exposed to SSRIs were also 10 times more likely to have been exposed to alcohol, making interpretation of the results difficult. Another problem is detecting these malformations, as thousands of pregnancies would need to be studied to determine a rare drug-induced defect. Since there are no concrete data linking SSRIs with cardiac malformations, the clinician should make a decision on an individual basis, weighing the pros and cons of changing or continuing medication at the risk of upsetting the mental state of the patient. Like TCAs, SSRIs are excreted in breast milk in small quantities. Paroxetine and sertraline, having shorter half-lives, are preferred in breastfeeding, whereas those with longer half-lives, such as citalopram and fluoxetine, are best avoided. In pregnancy and the post-partum period, it would seem that sertraline is a good choice from this class of antidepressants, as it is affordable, efficacious, well tolerated and has a safe side-effect profile.

Other antidepressants include the MAOIs and the newer antidepressants such as mirtazapine, venlafaxine, trazodone and duloxetine. MAOIs can make pregnancy-induced hypertension worse and may also be associated with congenital malformations. Due to potentially serious interactions with food, MAOIs should not be used if the mother is breastfeeding. If one sees a pregnant woman on an MAOI, then switching to a more favourable class should be discussed. A new antidepressant should not be started until 2 weeks have elapsed since stopping the MAOI. Venlafaxine and duloxetine are serotonin and noradrenaline reuptake inhibitors (SNRIs). Due to limited data on their safety, they should not be prescribed in pregnancy. Similarly, lack of use of mirtazapine and trazodone means they cannot be recommended for routine use, though early data do not suggest any increase in congenital malformations.

All antidepressants are associated with the 'neonatal adaptation syndrome', particularly when used in late pregnancy. This is a syndrome of the newborn infant. Symptoms include irritability, tachypnoea, temperature instability, low blood sugar and occasional seizures. This is thought to be due to drug withdrawal effects, though drug toxicity or alterations in infantile brain function may also be responsible. Reassuringly, this is of short duration, generally resolving within the first 2 weeks of life.

Examination practice: psychiatric disorders in pregnancy

Options for questions 6–8:

a PND

b personality disorder

c space occupying lesion

d post-traumatic stress disorder

e puerperal psychosis

f metabolic disorder

g baby blues

h anxiety disorder

i bipolar affective disorder.

Instructions: Each of the clinical scenarios below relate to women presenting in the post-partum period with psychiatric problems. For each patient, select the single most appropriate diagnosis from options a–i. Each option may be used once, more than once or not at all.

6 A midwife calls you to the home of a 24-year-old woman who gave birth to her first child 6 days ago. The woman tells you that a voice has told her that her husband is plotting to kill her and that the baby is not hers; rather, it is the child of the devil.

7 A 28-year-old woman, having given birth 4 days ago, presents to your surgery in a tearful state. She tells you that she feels emotionally unstable and anxious and has poor sleep. She has no negative feelings towards herself or the child. You review her a week later and she is back to her normal happy self.

8 After your surgery, the husband of a patient who had a baby 5 days ago calls you. He tells you that she seems to be uninterested in her child, is not eating and has poor sleep. She is constantly crying and has expressed a desire to kill herself by taking an overdose.

9 Mark the following statements as either true or false.

    a Depression is more common in pregnancy when the expectant mother is younger than 20 years old.

    b The use of antidepressant drugs in pregnancy is associated with a slightly increased risk of gestational diabetes and premature rupture of the membranes.

    c SSRI use is associated with infants large for their gestational age.

    d Exposure of the fetus to SSRIs, after 20 weeks, has been linked to an increased risk of persistent pulmonary hypertension of the newborn.

    e Electroconvulsive therapy (ECT) for severe depression is absolutely contraindicated in pregnancy due to the high risk of fetal burns.

10 Which of the following statements regarding bipolar disorder and its treatment in pregnancy are true?

    a In the immediate post-partum period, the risk of symptom recurrence is high in women with bipolar disorder.

    b The most common fetal cardiac malformation associated with lithium use in pregnancy is tetralogy of Fallot.

    c Lithium has been associated with an increased birthweight.

    d Lithium toxicity in the infant is associated with 'floppy baby syndrome', characterised by cyanosis and hypotonicity.

    e Lithium is not secreted in breast milk, making it a safe option if the mother chooses to breastfeed.

References

Anderson EL, Reti IM. ECT in pregnancy: a review of the literature from 1941 to 2007. *Psychosom Med.* 2009; **71**(2): 235–42.

Austin MP. To treat or not to treat: maternal depression, SSRI use in pregnancy and adverse neonatal effects. *Psychol Med.* 2006; **36**(12): 1663–70.

Collins S, Arulkumaran S, Hayes K, *et al.*, editors. *Oxford Handbook of Obstetrics and Gynaecology.* 2nd ed. Oxford: Oxford University Press; 2008.

Kimberly AY, Wisner KL, Stowe Z, *et al.* Management of bipolar disorder during pregnancy and the postpartum period. *Am J Psychiatry*. 2004; **161**(4): 608–20.

Oxfordshire and Buckinghamshire Mental Health NHS Foundation Trust. *Antidepressants: Safety in Pregnancy and Breast Feeding*. Medicines Information Bulletin. June 2010.

Stewart DE. Depression during pregnancy. *N Engl J Med*. 2011; **365**: 1605–11.

Wisner KL, Sit DK, Hanusa, BH, *et al*. Major depression and antidepressant treatment: impact on pregnancy and neonatal outcomes. *Am J Psychiatry*. 2009; **166**(5): 557–66.

Pregnancy and sexually transmitted infections

A 22-year-old woman presents to you during a busy morning surgery. She seems quite guarded as she tells you that her period is 2 weeks late and a pregnancy test carried out the day before was positive. You cautiously congratulate her. She tells you that she has a new partner of 3 months and is generally happy about the pregnancy. This is her first pregnancy. As you talk to her about the various aspects of a healthy pregnancy you note that she remains distant. You politely enquire whether there is something else on her mind. She replies, 'Doctor, I have noticed some spots down below which are very sore.' As you examine her, you realise she is suffering from genital herpes. She asks whether they are likely to harm her baby.

Which of the following statements are true?

a Reassuring her that this is a self-limiting condition is the appropriate course of action.

b Advise the patient that a caesarean section is inevitable.

c Management of this patient will vary depending on whether this is primary or recurrent herpes.

d Offer her a termination due to the serious morbidity and mortality associated with neonatal herpes.

e Risk to the baby is greatest when genital herpes is acquired in the first trimester.

Answer: c

Genital herpes simplex virus (HSV) disease is on the rise in the UK. It is estimated that one in eight women have genital herpes in the UK. This makes it quite likely that one may come across women with the condition who are pregnant. Genital herpes is not only a source of great distress to the woman but also can have devastating effects on the newborn infant in the form of neonatal HSV infection caused by either HSV-1 or HSV-2. HSV-1 infection is increasingly recognised as a cause of genital herpes in the younger population and may be more transmissible to the neonate than HSV-2. The majority of neonatal infections will result from neonatal exposure to the virus in genital tract secretions during delivery. In utero transmission is considered very rare.

The first step is to ascertain whether the case is of primary or recurrent genital herpes, which may not be as easy as it sounds. In some cases, the woman will give a clear history of genital herpes, which may be corroborated by her notes. Alternatively, a previous infection may have been ignored or gone unnoticed due to non-specific symptoms. Studies have also shown that many primary cases of herpes infection are misdiagnosed by clinicians. It is not possible to distinguish between a primary or recurrent infection by clinical examination alone. The reason that differentiation is so important is that primary infection, acquired particularly in the third trimester, carries the highest risk of transmission to the child, causing neonatal herpes. Recurrent herpes in the mother is likely to have resulted in the development of maternal neutralising antibodies, hence reducing the risk of infection in the infant. For this reason, the diagnosis of suspected genital herpes should be confirmed by swabs taken from the base of the ulcer. If the lesion is vesicular, then it should be de-roofed and a swab of the fluid taken. This will normally require referral to a genitourinary specialist who, depending on local guidelines and facilities available, may subsequently confirm the diagnosis by viral culture or HSV DNA detection via real-time PCR. This latter method has higher HSV detection rates.

Women with a history of recurrent genital herpes can be reassured that the risk of neonatal transmission and herpes infection is very low. There is also no evidence that their condition will be made worse by pregnancy. They should be counselled towards a vaginal delivery. Opinions differ as to how such women should be managed if they develop HSV lesions at onset of labour. Recurrent genital herpes with active lesions at labour onset is associated with a small risk (1%–3%) to the baby of neonatal herpes if it is delivered vaginally. This needs to be offset against the risk of caesarean section to the mother. One American study suggests that if all women with recurrent genital herpes with active lesions at labour were to have a caesarean section, then the number of patients that would need to be treated to prevent one case of herpes-related mortality or morbidity would be 1583. Despite this, most mothers, with active genital herpes at the onset of labour in the USA, are recommended to have a caesarean section, advice probably influenced by the medico-legal risk. There is evidence that 400 mg of acyclovir taken three times per day in the last 4 weeks of pregnancy is beneficial as it reduces the risk of developing a recurrence of HSV at delivery and the chance of a caesarean section having to be performed. Whether prophylactic antiviral treatment reduces the risk of neonatal HSV infection is unclear.

A woman presenting in pregnancy with primary genital herpes will need to be referred to a specialist genitourinary clinic for the investigations described. The patient should be screened for other sexually transmitted infections (STIs), in particular for human immunodeficiency virus (HIV) as co-infection results in increased replication of both viruses. She should be treated with acyclovir, either orally or intravenously, depending on her clinical condition. Although there is no evidence of teratogenicity, acyclovir is unlicensed for use in pregnancy. If the presentation is in the first or second trimester, the pregnancy should be managed expectantly with the hope of delivering vaginally. She may also be treated with prophylactic acyclovir from 36 weeks onwards to reduce the risk of developing genital lesions at delivery, although evidence of benefit of this is lacking. All women developing primary genital HSV in the third trimester should be referred to an obstetrician to discuss operative delivery due to the high risk of neonatal transmission. The risk of transmission is at its highest if the episode of primary infection occurs in the final 6 weeks of pregnancy. Invasive procedures should be avoided if the woman chooses to have a vaginal delivery. Either way, a neonatologist should be informed of the birth to assess the child, take appropriate swabs and samples, and decide if antiviral treatment needs to be started.

Examination practice: STIs in pregnancy

Options for questions 11–13:

a   metronidazole 2 g single dose

b   benzathine penicillin G 2.4 MU intramuscularly

c   azithromycin 1 g orally as single dose

d   lamivudine 100 mg daily

e   options c and h combined

f   acyclovir 800 mg five times per day for 7 days

g   options a and c combined

h   ceftriaxone 500 mg intramuscularly

i   cefixime 400 mg orally.

Instructions: Questions 11–13 refer to women presenting with STIs. From the list, choose the most appropriate (first-line) treatment for each scenario. Each option may be used once, more than once or not at all.

11   A 30-year-old woman develops a painless ulcer on her vulva. Examination of fluid from the ulcer confirms syphilis.

12   A 26-year-old woman presents with dysuria and a mild vaginal discharge. An endocervical swab confirms gonorrhoea.

13 An 18-year-old university student requests contraception on a routine visit. An opportunistic chlamydia screen is positive.

14 Which of the following statements are true regarding neonatal herpes infection?

    a Postnatal transmission of virus to the neonate may occur from orolabial lesions.

    b The highest fatality rate with neonatal herpes is associated with cutaneous disease, which accounts for 45% of clinical manifestations.

    c Intravenous acyclovir has been shown to reduce mortality when given to infants with CNS and disseminated disease.

    d High doses of acyclovir are associated with transient neutropenia in the treated infant.

    e Cutaneous HSV infection in the newborn responds well to topical acyclovir.

15 Which of the following statements are true regarding HIV infection in pregnancy?

    a Breastfeeding is associated with a twofold increase in the rate of HIV transmission.

    b All pregnant women should be offered screening for HIV at 36 weeks because all transmission from mother to child occurs after this.

    c In mothers who have HIV and are not taking antiretroviral therapy with a detectable viral load, elective caesarean section is of clear benefit in reducing vertical transmission.

    d Mothers with HIV should be encouraged to breastfeed early to boost the child's immune system against HIV.

    e A negative HIV antibody test at 18 months confirms that the child is unaffected.

References

Bignell C, FitzGerald M. UK national guideline for the management of gonorrhoea in adults, 2011. *Int J STD AIDS.* 2011; **22**(10): 541–7.

Corey L, Wald A. Maternal and neonatal herpes simplex virus infections. *N Engl J Med.* 2009; **361**: 1376–85.

Foley E. Herpes in pregnancy: how to avoid neonatal transmission. *Br J Sex Med.* 2010; **33**(2): 4–7.

Hollier LM, Wendel GD. Third trimester antiviral prophylaxis for preventing maternal genital herpes simplex virus (HSV) recurrences and neonatal infection. *Cochrane Database Sys Rev.* 2008; **23**(1): CD004946.

Horner P, Boag F. *2006 UK National Guideline for the Management of Genital Tract Infection with Chlamydia Trachomatis.* London: British Association for Sexual Health and HIV; n.d. Available at: www.bashh.org/documents/61/61.pdf (accessed 11 January 2012).

Kingston M, French P, Goh B, *et al.* UK national guidelines on the management of syphilis 2008. *Int J STD AIDS.* 2008; **19**(11): 729–40.

RGOG. *Management of Genital Herpes in Pregnancy.* Green-top Guideline No. 30. London: Guidelines and Audit Committee of the RCOG; March 2009.

RGOG. *Management of HIV in Pregnancy.* Green-top Guideline No. 39. London: Guidelines and Audit Committee of the RCOG; March 2009. Available at: www.rcog.org.uk/files/rcog-corp/uploaded-files/GtG_no_39_HIV_in_pregnancy_June_2010_v2011.pdf (accessed 3 March 2012).

Pregnancy and obesity

A 28-year-old receptionist comes to you for pre-pregnancy counselling. You note that she is generally fit and well. Her current medication is orlistat 120 mg three times per day, which was started by one of your colleagues 6 months ago. The following details were listed in her file at her last visit with the practice nurse.

Thinking about getting pregnant. Struggling with her weight.
> *Weight 85 kg*
> *Height 155 cm*
> *BP 110/70*
> *BMI 35*
> *Advised to see GP*

She is keen to know whether she should continue with her exercise regime at the gym. She would also like to know if she needs to take any additional precautions due to her weight.

Which of the following statements are true?
a   Orlistat is known to cause cardiac malformations in the growing fetus.
b   Exercise is best avoided in pregnancy.

c   There is an increased risk of developing gestational diabetes in pregnancy in obese women.

d   Maternal body mass index (BMI) has a strong correlation with the increased incidence of haemolysis, elevated liver enzymes and low platelet count (HELLP) syndrome.

e   Caesarean section rates are greater in obese women than in non-obese women.

f   There is evidence that exercise in obese women reduces the risk of developing gestational diabetes mellitus.

Answer: c, e and f

The growing pandemic of obesity is a well-known issue. The last *Health Survey for England* showed that one in four adults and one in ten children between the ages of 2 and 15 years old are classified as obese. According to the Department of Health, the estimated cost to the NHS is around £4 billion per year. The problem does not end there, as it is a problem on the increase. If the current trend continues, it is estimated that half of the adult and one quarter of the child population will be obese by 2050. It is therefore not surprising that we deal with more pregnant women who are classified as obese. This is a worrying trend, as the obese gravida is associated with far greater risks when compared with her non-obese counterpart. Obesity is a risk to the pregnant mother, the fetus and the newborn. In the mother, obesity increases the risk of gestational diabetes, maternal hypertension and pre-eclampsia. There is also a greater risk of fetal macrosomia, trauma to mother and child at birth and fetal malformations. Post-partum complications include an increased rate of delayed wound healing following caesarean section, post-partum haemorrhage, infection and thrombosis. There is also increasing evidence to suggest that 'in utero programming' increases the risk of developing lifelong complications such as diabetes and heart disease in children born to obese mothers. It is therefore imperative that health professionals are well equipped at the point of contact to help individuals such as those mentioned in the case discussed.

This case is an example of the ideal scenario in which pre-pregnancy counselling is sought. It is at this stage that the imperativeness of weight loss must be reiterated. Obesity is strongly linked to increased caloric intake in conjunction with very little energy expenditure. This should be discussed with patients in the hope of encouraging a sensible diet and increasing their exercise levels. Patients often underestimate their caloric intake. A food diary over the course of 2–3 weeks is generally an eye opener for both the doctor and patient, as the latter realises that their diet is probably not as good as they thought. A diet high in fibre, lean protein and complex carbohydrates should be encouraged. Cakes, sweets and biscuits should be strongly discouraged. Patients with poor understanding of their diet or those struggling to lose weight should be referred to a dietician. Many people consider 'work' to be exercise, but this may not necessarily be the case. However, there is no reason why aspects of work cannot be made into exercise. Patients should be encouraged to take daily, moderate, aerobic exercise for at least 30 minutes. Encourage patients to take a brisk walk that gets them slightly puffing. Patients will find it easier to incorporate this in to their day-to-day activities, as the 'walk back from the station' or the 'trip to the shops for a pint of milk' can become their daily dose of exercise. Brisk stair climbing can also work for those stuck indoors.

The level of exercise permissible in pregnancy often comes up in a consultation. The Royal College of Obstetricians and Gynaecologists (RCOG) has some guidelines available on their website under the title 'Recreational exercise and pregnancy'. This is a good resource to refer to when advising patients. Pregnant women should be advised that aerobic exercise, such as running, brisk walking and swimming, is permissible and recommended in pregnancy. However, the idea is not to reach peak levels of fitness. Women should be advised to avoid getting too hot, to drink plenty of water, stretch prior to starting exercise and avoid exercises that involve lying on their back, particularly after 16 weeks, due to the risk of hypotension from aortic compression. Contact sports and scuba diving should be discouraged. If they are short of breath when talking after an exercise session, they are probably exercising too hard and should reduce their exercise levels. As pregnancy progresses, the level of exercise will also need to be reduced. Exercise advice should be tailored to the individual. Someone who has never done exercise before will obviously need to follow a different regime from a seasoned athlete. The aim in pregnancy is to limit weight gain rather than lose weight. Patients should be told that exercise in pregnancy helps relieve tiredness, constipation, nausea, back pain and leg swelling. Thirty minutes of exercise a day is not associated with any adverse outcomes. However, high levels of exercise (>270 minutes a week) have been associated with a low, yet significant, increase in the risk of severe pre-eclampsia.

Orlistat, a lipase inhibitor, is licensed for use in obesity. It is currently recommended in those with a BMI >30 kg/m^2; however, it can be prescribed to those with a BMI of 28 kg/m^2 if they have other pre-existing risk factors for heart disease such as diabetes, high cholesterol or hypertension. It works by preventing fat absorption in the gut. As a result, the unabsorbed fat makes its way to the rectum and will usually manifest itself as an oily leakage, a symptom that can be very troublesome for those with a high fat content in their diet. It therefore works like a diet modifier: patients notice which foods make their rectal leakage worse and consequently stop eating them. Others, however, just stop taking the drug. Although animal studies have shown orlistat to be safe in pregnancy, lack of clinical trials in humans means it is not recommended in pregnancy. It is also to be avoided in breastfeeding. Centrally acting appetite suppressants, such as sibutramine, have been withdrawn due to their adverse side effects.

Due to the adverse outcomes associated with obesity in the mother and child, bariatric surgery may be considered in the most extreme cases. The National Institute for Health and Clinical Excellence (NICE) guidelines set out who should be eligible for bariatric surgery. Individuals with either a BMI of >40 kg/m^2 or a BMI >35 kg/m^2 with other co-morbidities such as diabetes or hypertension, the control of which is likely to improve with surgery, may be considered.

Greater effort should be made to counsel women early in the prenatal period to minimise the risk to mother and child in later pregnancy. Care will be multidimensional and multidisciplined. Primary care physicians are at the front line of this care and need to be well equipped to manage this group of patients.

Examination practice: routine antenatal care

Options for questions 16–18:

a 4 weeks

b 12 weeks

c 10–13 weeks

d 18–20 weeks

e 28 and 34 weeks

f 26 and 32 weeks

g 37 weeks

h 40 weeks

i 42 weeks.

Instructions: Each of the following clinical scenarios relate to antenatal appointments. For each scenario, select the single most appropriate time in the antenatal period when it should take place from the options listed. Each option may be used once, more than once or not at all.

16 External cephalic version (ECV) for breech presentation in a multiparous woman.

17 Detailed USS to determine congenital anomalies.

18 A 6-week pregnant, fit and well woman asks you how long into her pregnancy she should continue taking folic acid supplements.

19 On routine clinical examination of a pregnant woman, which of the following would be considered abnormal?

    a A dark pigmented line running all the way from the xiphisternum to the suprapubic area, through the umbilicus.

   b   An increase in lumbar lordosis on spinal examination.

   c   Abdominally palpable uterus at 12 weeks.

   d   A symphysis–fundal height (SFH) of 28 cm at 32 weeks' gestation.

   e   Flattening or eversion of the umbilicus.

20 Which of the following blood tests is not done routinely at the booking visit?

   a   Full blood count (FBC).

   b   Syphilis screen.

   c   Rubella antibodies.

   d   Blood group and antibody screen.

   e   Glucose tolerance test.

References

Collins S, Arulkumaran S, Hayes K, *et al.*, editors. *Oxford Handbook of Obstetrics and Gynaecology*. 2nd ed. Oxford: Oxford University Press; 2008.

Duckitt K. Exercise during pregnancy. Eat for one, exercise for two. *BMJ*. 2011; **343**: 1129.

Gunatilake RP, Jordan HP. Obesity and pregnancy: clinical management of the obese gravida. *Am J Obstet Gynaecol*. 2011; **204**(2): 106–19.

RGOG. *External Cephalic Version (ECV) and Reducing the Incidence of Breech Presentation*. Green-top Guideline No. 20a. London: Guidelines and Audit Committee of the RCOG; December 2006. Available at: www.rcog.org.uk/files/rcog-corp/uploaded-files/GT20aExternalCephalicVersion.pdf (accessed 6 March 2012).

RGOG. *Recreational Exercise and Pregnancy: information for you*. London: RGOG; September 2006. Available at: www.rcog.org.uk/files/rcog-corp/uploaded-files/PIRecreationalExercise2006.pdf (accessed 6 March 2012).

RCOG. *Ultrasound Screening*. London: RCOG; 2000. Available at: www.rcog.org.uk/womens-health/clinical-guidance/ultrasound-screening (accessed 30 January 2012).

The National Health Service (NHS) Information Centre Lifestyles Statistics. *Statistics on Obesity, Physical Activity and Diet: England, 2010*. Leeds: NHS

Information Centre for Health and Social Care; 2010. Available at: www. ic.nhs.uk/webfiles/publications/opad10/Statistics_on_Obesity_Physical_ Activity_and_Diet_England_2010.pdf (accessed 30 January 2012).

World Health Organization (WHO). *Definition and Diagnosis of Diabetes Mellitus and Intermediate Hyperglycaemia: report of a WHO/IDF consultation.* Geneva: WHO; 2006. Available at: www.who.int/diabetes/publications/Definition%20 and%20diagnosis%20of%20diabetes_new.pdf (accessed 11 January 2012).

Abdominal masses and surgery

A 32-year-old patient presents to you in clinic. She informs you that she has irregular periods and has not had one for 3 months. She felt her tummy getting larger so she did a pregnancy test and according to the strip she is 6 weeks pregnant. She is a gravida 3 para 2. She tells you that she thinks she is more than 6 weeks pregnant, as her tummy feels larger than it did at 6 weeks in her previous pregnancies. In fact, she has felt her tummy getting bigger for at least 3 months. You offer to examine her and find a mass in her abdomen, equivalent to 12 weeks' gestation. However, it feels different from a fetus and appears to originate from the right adnexa. You explain your findings and send her for a USS to confirm. The sonographer's report is as follows.

Complex mass originating from the right adnexa. Approximately 10 cm in diameter. Appears cystic. Difficult to perform tissue characterisation. Suggest further imaging.

Viable intrauterine sac of 6 weeks' gestation also noted.

Which of the following statements is true?

a   Ultrasound was a poor choice of imaging in this case due to its poor sensitivity and specificity in assessing adnexal masses.

b   Tumour markers such as CA-125 would be very useful in the diagnosis of the mass in this case.

c   Functional cysts account for the majority of adnexal masses in pregnancy.

d   Laparoscopy is contraindicated in pregnancy due to the risk of fetal acidosis.

e   Observation is an acceptable form of management for certain adnexal masses in pregnancy, as up to two-thirds of ovarian masses that appear benign will either resolve spontaneously or regress in size during the course of the pregnancy.

f   Pregnant women undergoing surgery in pregnancy are at an increased risk of delivering prematurely compared with pregnant women not undergoing surgery.

Answer: c, e and f

Adnexal masses in pregnancy are generally either picked up as in this case or during the routine 12- or 20-week USS. Rarely, they may be discovered during labour due to the mother having evaded the routine surveillance programme. In the latter scenario, they can have quite dramatic consequences, as these masses are at an increased risk of torsion, rupturing or obstructing labour. Hence, early identification and monitoring are vital.

The incidence of various adnexal masses in pregnancy is similar to their incidence outside of pregnancy. Thus, functional cysts, such as a persistent corpus luteum, can account for up to one in six of all cystic adnexal masses. Dermoid cyst, another benign mass, is also a common diagnosis in pregnancy. Ovarian malignancies of low or high malignant potential account for around 1%–8% of adnexal masses in pregnancy.

Clinically, an adnexal mass is difficult to differentiate from the more frequently occurring mass of the uterine cavity – fibroids. Therefore, an imaging technique is required that is safe in pregnancy. Such a technique needs to successfully identify the mass and suggest its malignant potential so that an informed decision may be made regarding management; ultrasound scanning fits this bill perfectly. Many studies have shown that ultrasound is very effective in differentiating the morphology and determining the malignant potential of the mass. Doppler techniques can also be added to ultrasound scanning to look for the different blood flow patterns in benign and malignant masses, although studies have yet to verify any additional diagnostic benefit this may contribute. The additional safety of ultrasound scanning to the mother and the fetus makes it the perfect and preferred method for radiological assessment of the mass.

There will be cases, like the one discussed here, in which ultrasound scanning will be unable to fully determine the nature of the mass. In such cases, computed tomography (CT) scans and magnetic resonance imaging (MRI) are of benefit. Both are considered safe in pregnancy, but the former is associated with a high dose of radiation to both the mother and the fetus. If contrast material is used, then the patient should be made aware of the risk of it crossing the placental barrier; however, the effects of this on the fetus are unclear.

Tumour markers such as CA-125 are not very helpful in diagnosing the nature of the mass, as they are raised in a whole host of benign and malignant disease processes. However, they do have a role in disease monitoring, as a rising CA-125 may indicate increased tumour activity.

As with most things in medicine, opinions regarding management are divided. Broadly speaking, management may be observational – that is, 'watch and wait' – or surgical. Advocates of the watch and wait method argue that most adnexal masses detected in pregnancy will spontaneously resolve, thus, aggressive surgical management will not be necessary. Smaller, simple-looking masses picked up earlier in pregnancy are more likely to resolve on their own. Another factor in support of observation is the fact that pregnant women undergoing surgery are at a greater risk of delivering prematurely.

Surgery in pregnancy for an adnexal mass may be via laparotomy or laparoscopy, the former being the more traditional method. Both methods have their pros and cons. Since there are no head-to-head studies, advocates of each argue their corner vigorously. Laparotomy is tried and tested and has a very good safety profile. There are no concerns, as there may be in the laparoscopic approach, regarding the effects of introducing air into the peritoneum on the fetus, the risk of damage to the fetus by the trocar or other surgical instruments or the potential of fetal acidosis. However, laparotomy is associated with a longer hospital stay, greater use of analgesics and longer recovery period than laparoscopy. Many studies have looked at the safety profile of laparoscopy in managing adnexal masses in pregnancy and it is no longer considered contraindicated in pregnancy. In the presence of a skilled operator, laparoscopy may be considered the preferable method. The optimal time for laparoscopy is at 16–20 weeks. One must bear in mind that the mentioned increased risk of prematurity in women undergoing surgery is irrespective of the surgical method used.

Therefore, management is determined by a number of factors. Patient wishes should always be considered and any delay in surgery should be balanced by the risks of mechanical obstruction of labour, torsion, rupture and delaying treatment of potential malignant disease.

Examination practice: gynaecological and obstetric surgery

Options for questions 21–23:

a   ovarian electrocautery

b   Burch colposuspension

c   Wertheim's procedure

d   posterior colporrhaphy

e   colposcopy

f   cervical cerclage

g   cystourethroplasty

h   Marshall–Marchetti–Krantz procedure

i   large loop excision of the transformation zone (LLETZ).

Instructions: Each of the clinical scenarios that follow relate to women requesting surgery for various gynaecological problems. For each patient, select the single most appropriate surgical management from the list of options. Each option may be used once, more than once or not at all.

21 A 60-year-old woman with stress incontinence would like surgery. On examination, there is no evidence of prolapse.

22 A 24-year-old Asian woman with polycystic ovarian syndrome (PCOS) seeks a surgical solution to her anovulation.

23 A 28-year-old woman with three previous second-trimester miscarriages, who has fallen pregnant again, seeks to improve her chances of a successful pregnancy.

24 In the management of women with third- and fourth-degree perineal tears, which of the following statements is true?
    a Repair should be carried out in the labour room under local anaesthesia.
    b Endoanal ultrasound has no role to play in management.
    c Laxatives should be avoided, as they contribute to wound dehiscence.
    d All women should be offered physiotherapy and advised to perform pelvic floor exercises.
    e There is no role for antibiotics.

25 Choose the single most correct statement regarding uterine fibroids and their management.
    a There is strong evidence supporting intervention in women with asymptomatic fibroids.
    b An enlarging abdominal mass is the most common symptom of fibroids.
    c There is a tendency for fibroids to regress after the menopause.
    d Fibroid embolisation is the treatment of choice in pregnancy.
    e Fibroid embolisation is associated with minimal post-procedure pain.

References

Final report of the Medical Research Council/Royal College of Obstetricians and Gynaecologists multicentre randomised trial of cervical cerclage. MRC/RCOG working party on cervical cerclage. *Br J Obstet Gynaecol.* 1993; **100**(6): 516–23.

Gjønnaess H. Late endocrine effects of ovarian electrocautery in women with polycystic ovary syndrome. *Fertil Steril.* 1998; **69**(4): 697–701.

Goodwin SC, Spies JB. Uterine fibroid embolization. *N Engl J Med.* 2009; **361**(7): 690–7.

Hoover K, Jenkins TR. Evaluation and management of adnexal mass in pregnancy. *Am J Obstet Gynecol.* 2011; **205**(2): 97–103.

Lapitan MC, Cody DJ, Grant AM. Open retropubic colposuspension for urinary incontinence in women. *Cochrane Database Syst Rev.* 2005: **2**; CD002912.

RGOG. *The Investigation and Treatment of Couples with Recurrent Miscarriage.* Green-top Guideline No. 17. London: Guidelines and Audit Committee of the RCOG; May 2011. Available at: www.rcog.org.uk/files/rcog-corp/GTG17recurrentmiscarriage.pdf (accessed 6 March 2012).

RGOG. *The Management of Third- and Fourth-Degree Perineal Tears.* Green-top Guideline No. 29. London: Guidelines and Audit Committee of the RCOG; January 2007. Available at: www.rcog.org.uk/files/rcog-corp/GTG2911022011.pdf (accessed 6 March 2012).

RGOG. *Surgical Treatment of Urodynamic Stress Incontinence.* Green-top Guideline No. 35. London: Guidelines and Audit Committee of the RCOG; January 2003.

Rogers RG. Urinary stress incontinence in women. *N Engl J Med.* 2008; **358**(10): 1029–36.

Premenstrual syndrome

A 22-year-old female patient sees you in your surgery. You scan her notes and see that she saw one of your colleagues 6 months ago for ongoing problems with stress and irritability. Her symptoms would typically begin 2 weeks prior to her menstruation and ease considerably with the onset of bleeding. She would be 'a different person' for the next 2 weeks until the '2 weeks from hell' would begin again. She reported headaches, breast swelling and discomfort, mood swings, inability to concentrate and feeling excessively tired. The severity of her symptoms would leave her tearful at times and prone to bursts of anger, the recipient of which would be her poor boyfriend. Your colleague, after ascertaining that there were no contraindications, started her on a combined oral contraceptive pill (COCP). He recommended a 6-monthly review and asked her to complete the Daily Record of Severity of Problems, a questionnaire logging her symptoms, for months 1–2 and 5–6 of her treatment. She presents today and bursts into tears, saying that her relationship is on the brink of breakdown due to her symptoms. You look at her completed questionnaire and note that her scores are very high for the latter part of the cycle.

Which of the following statements are true?

a There is strong evidence for the efficacy of levonorgestrel-based oral contraceptives in the management of the premenstrual syndrome (PMS).

b PMS is more common in women of higher academic achievement.

c PMS is caused by a pathological imbalance of ovarian hormones.

d Due to the availability of highly effective alternatives, bilateral oopherectomy is no longer a valid option in the management of PMS.

e Gonadotrophin-releasing hormone (GnRH) analogues work by inducing a state similar to the menopause hence controlling symptoms of PMS.

Answer: e

'PMS' refers to the distressing symptoms that recur in the luteal phase of the menstrual cycle. These may be physical, behavioural, psychological or a combination of all three. The symptoms will usually have resolved by the end of menstruation. However, 'premenstrual exaggeration' may occur when there is incomplete relief from the symptoms after the end of menstruation, resulting in persistent low-grade residual symptoms. PMS is characterised by the significant impact it has on patients' day-to-day life. It is more common in women of low academic achievement and in the obese.

When women initially present with symptoms suggestive of PMS, it is good practice to get them to start a symptom diary. This can simply be subjective scoring of the day, on a scale of 1 to 10, through the course of the month. A more formalised scoring system such as the Daily Record of Severity of Problems may also be used. This is a more comprehensive questionnaire asking patients to rate their physical, behavioural and psychological symptoms on a scale of 1 to 6. Over the course of 2 months, this should give a good idea of the pattern and severity of the patient's symptoms.

There is no consensus as to how PMS should be managed, so in most cases it will mean trying various treatment modalities individually or in combination. Current opinion is that PMS is caused by normal ovarian function rather than an aberration in hormonal balance. Neurotransmitters such as serotonin and gamma-amino butyric acid (GABA) are believed to play a role in causing the symptoms of PMS. Evidence for the deficiency of progesterone as a cause of PMS is very limited; thus, it is not surprising that treatment with progesterone generally has a poor outcome.

Primary care physicians manage most cases of PMS. Available treatment modalities include the following.

- Lifestyle changes. There is some evidence that moderate aerobic exercise may help improve the symptoms of PMS. Other measures may include reduction in alcohol and caffeine intake. A diet with a low glycaemic index may also be beneficial.

- Complementary therapies. Many physicians may feel uncomfortable referring patients to a complementary medicine practitioner due to the lack of evidence in their benefit. However, there is some evidence that some complementary treatments may be of a small benefit; hence, a multifaceted approach to the problem can include their use. Vitamin D and calcium compounds, vitamin B6 and extract of the fruit of *Vitex agnus-castus*, the chaste tree, have the best data available amongst the dizzying array of vitamins and potions available. Evening primrose oil may improve the symptoms of cyclical mastalgia associated with PMS. High doses of vitamin B6 (200 mg or more daily) are associated with a risk of peripheral neuropathy, requiring caution in their use. The usual dose of vitamin B6 in PMS is 50–100 mg daily.

- Psychological therapies. The RCOG recommends the routine use of cognitive behavioural therapy (CBT) in the treatment of PMS. Although it may be associated with a slower response, it may be more effective in maintaining remission for a longer period. The main issue with CBT is problems accessing the service. If available, it should be offered as one of the first options, provided the patient is willing to try it.

- Hormonal therapies. The use of hormone-based therapies is predicated on the understanding that disrupting the normal cycle should suppress symptoms of PMS. This can be justified by the phenomenon of improvement of PMS symptoms during pregnancy and the postmenopausal phase. COCPs, though widely used, have not proved very effective in placebo-controlled trials. Newer COCPs containing drosperinone or norgestimate (e.g. Yasmin® and Cilest®, respectively) as their progesterone component have shown some promise in controlling PMS symptoms, thus, may be used in preference to the older COCPs. Oestrogen may also be delivered by a patch or an implant; 100 mcg is the preferred dose. In patients with an intact uterus, cyclical progesterone must also be given. If the oral preparation exacerbates PMS symptoms, then a levonorgestrel-releasing intrauterine system (Mirena® coil) may be inserted.

- Antidepressants. There is good evidence for the use of SSRIs in the treatment of PMS. The RCOG recommends them as a first-line treatment due to their proven efficacy. SNRIs, such as venlafaxine, are also known to be effective but have a less favourable tolerability profile, rendering them second choice. SSRIs may be given continuously, cyclically during the luteal phase of the menstrual cycle or with the onset of symptoms. The advantage of the latter two methods is that they are not associated with withdrawal effects on cessation of treatment. Fluoxetine (20–60 mg daily) and sertraline (50–150 mg daily) are the SSRIs with the most evidence for their use. Higher doses of these are generally associated with greater side effects and potential discontinuation of therapy. A reasonable approach would be to start with the lowest possible dose and increase if necessary until symptom control is achieved. SSRIs and SNRIs may be combined with hormonal therapies safely, though evidence of their efficacy in combination is lacking. There is also some evidence to support the use of TCAs such as clomipramine and nortriptyline for the treatment of PMS.
- Others. Danazol, an androgenic steroid, disrupts the hormone cycle. It can be used at a dose of 200 mg twice per day. However, its use is limited due to its potential virilising effects in the female. Anxiolytics such as alprazolam and buspirone may also have some benefit, but their routine use is not recommended. Similarly, luteal-phase spironolactone may also have some benefit in improving mood and somatic symptoms of PMS.

Other treatments, usually the domain of secondary care, include GnRH analogues (which can be considered chemical oophorectomies, as they induce a menopausal state in the patient) and, in the most severe cases, surgical removal of the ovaries; that is, an oophorectomy. It is only when these complex options are being considered that a referral to secondary care is indicated.

Examination practice: menstruation-related problems

Options for questions 26–28:

a   Asherman's syndrome

b   Laurence–Moon syndrome

c   Sheehan's syndrome

d   haematocolpos

e   PCOS

f   premature ovarian failure

g   Turner's syndrome

h   Perrault syndrome

i   Swyer syndrome.

Instructions: Each of the clinical scenarios that follow relate to women presenting with amenorrhoea due to different underlying problems. For each patient, select the most likely diagnosis from the list of options provided.

26   A 16-year-old girl presents with her mother, never having had periods. You note that she is of short stature, has a short, webbed neck and a scutiform thorax.

27   A 30-year-old woman presents with secondary amenorrhoea. In the past, she had two dilatation and curettage procedures under gynaecologists for heavy periods. A recent hysteroscopy report noted uterine occlusion with synechiae.

28   A 16-year-old girl comes to your surgery with primary amenorrhoea. She has been suffering from cyclical lower abdominal pain over the last

few months. You note that she has good breast growth for her age and has pubic and axillary hair. She has an abdominal mass rising from the pelvis.

29 Which of the following statements regarding menorrhagia are true?
a Menorrhagia is associated only with ovulatory cycles.
b Tranexamic acid, an antifibrinolytic, is effective in reducing blood flow in the management of menorrhagia.
c Menorrhagia is the most common cause of iron deficiency anaemia in the Western world.
d In women with menorrhagia with an underlying bleeding disorder, the most common cause is haemophilia.
e The levonorgestrel-releasing intrauterine system (Mirena coil) is an effective alternative to surgery in the management of menorrhagia.

30 Which of the following statements regarding primary ovarian insufficiency (premature menopause) is false?
a The underlying cause in the majority of cases remains unknown.
b Five to ten per cent of women with a diagnosis of primary ovarian insufficiency will conceive and deliver a child.
c Primary ovarian insufficiency may be familial, with an affected first-degree relative in approximately 15% of cases.
d Primary ovarian insufficiency with a strong family history of intellectual disability may suggest a mutation in the FMR1 (fragile X mental retardation 1) gene.
e The presence of ovarian antibodies is highly sensitive and specific for diagnosing autoimmune primary ovarian failure.

References

Anthony J, Kaye P. *Notes for the DRCOG*. 4th ed. London: Churchill Livingstone; 2001.

Cecutti A. Case report: haematocolpos with imperforate hymen. *Can Med Assoc J.* 1964; **90**(25): 1420–1.

Draper R, Tidy C. *Turner Syndrome*. Leeds: Patient.co.uk; 2012. Available at: www.patient.co.uk/doctor/Turner's-Syndrome.htm (accessed 30 January 2012).

Grady-Weliky TA. Premenstrual dysphoric disorder. *N Engl J Med.* 2003; **348**(5): 433–8.

Nelson LM. Primary ovarian insufficiency. *N Engl J Med.* 2009; **360**(6): 606–14.

Prentice A. Fortnightly review: medical management of menorrhagia. *BMJ.* 1999; **319**: 1343–5.

RGOG. *Management of Premenstrual Syndrome*. Green-top Guideline No. 48. London: Guidelines and Audit Committee of the RCOG; December 2007. Available at: www.rcog.org.uk/files/rcog-corp/uploaded-files/GT48 ManagementPremensturalSyndrome.pdf (accessed 7 March 2012).

Welsh VK, O'Brien PMS. How to handle premenstrual syndrome in primary care. *Br J Sex Med.* 2009; **32**(4): 4–7.

Bacterial vaginosis

Your next patient is a 40-year-old woman. You take a cursory look at her notes and notice that she has seen various colleagues at the surgery about a recurring vaginal discharge. She describes the discharge as grey in colour and having a fishy odour. A recent vaginal swab confirmed the presence of clue cells and a diagnosis of bacterial vaginosis (BV) was made. Since then, she has had three courses of metronidazole, which have provided only short periods of relief. She is married with three children and lives with her husband, who has been her only sexual contact in the last 20 years. She comes in complaining of the recurrence and wanting 'a referral to a specialist to find out what is going on'.

Which of the following statements are false?

a   BV is a sexually transmitted disease.
b   The change in the *Lactobacillus* population of the vagina and resultant pH change occurs only in BV.
c   BV is associated with an increased risk of spontaneous miscarriage in pregnancy.
d   In BV, the vaginal pH is below 4.5.
e   BV is rare in children.

f   Probiotics with various strains of lactobacilli have been shown to be effective in reducing infection.

Answer: a, b and d

Despite being one of the most common causes of vaginal discharge, BV is a poorly understood condition. BV is associated with an overgrowth of anaerobic organisms that results in a reduction in the normal *Lactobacillus* population of the vagina. The ensuing reduction in lactate production results in a rise in the vaginal pH. This change in bacterial flora and rise in vaginal pH is not unique to BV. Aerobic vaginitis (AV) is a separate entity from BV that causes similar changes in the vaginal microflora and a rise in vaginal pH. As its name suggests, the vagina is predominantly colonised by aerobic organisms, originating from the gut, such as *Escherichia coli*, group B *Streptococcus* and *Staphylococcus aureus*. Unlike BV, AV is usually associated with an inflammation reaction. BV tends to present as an increased vaginal discharge, typically with a fishy odour. AV will also present with an increased vaginal discharge, typically non-malodorous, with burning, stinging and, occasionally, dyspareunia. Both AV and BV are important, not only due to the significant impact they can have on a woman's health, but also due to the adverse effects they may have on pregnancy, such as spontaneous miscarriage and preterm birth. AV is mentioned here to make the reader aware of it as a possible differential diagnosis in vaginal discharge. The high prevalence of BV has resulted in other vaginal flora not being described so often, resulting in their possible neglect. The remainder of this case will deal with the management of BV specifically.

BV is most common in women of childbearing age and may also be seen in the postmenopausal phase; it is rare in children. BV is not classified as a sexually transmitted disease. However, it is more common in women having sex or in those having changed a sexual partner.

Many consider Gram staining the gold standard for diagnosis; however, microscopic evaluation of vaginal fluid is widely used and accepted as very accurate. The microbiologist will comment on the presence of clue cells suggestive of BV. Adding potassium hydroxide to vaginal fluid results in the release of a fishy odour. Known as the 'whiff test', this also suggests BV.

The most important step in management is patient awareness. Patients should be told that this is not a STI. About half the women with BV will be blissfully unaware of the infection due to the lack of symptoms. Vaginal douching should be discouraged. Women should avoid excessive cleaning of the vagina and excessive use of bath oils, scented washing products, antiseptics and harsh detergents for washing underwear. The purpose of these measures is to avoid disruption of the normal vaginal flora.

It is not necessary that all women be treated with antibiotics, as BV may remit spontaneously. However, one should be aware that, apart from the mentioned risk to the fetus, BV increases the risk of acquiring STIs, such as genital HSV and HIV, post-termination endometritis and infection post-hysterectomy. These added risks should be considered when deciding whether treating with antibiotics is appropriate. Antibiotics may be taken orally or applied vaginally. Oral metronidazole seems to be the most widely used antibiotic for BV; 400–500 mg twice a day for 5–7 days is the recommended regime. Metronidazole is also available in a 0.75% strength gel. One applicator should be inserted vaginally every night for 5 nights. Oral metronidazole commonly causes a metallic taste in the mouth and stomach pains. These symptoms are more pronounced if a 2 g stat dose of metronidazole is used to treat the BV. It is also well known for causing a pronounced disulfiram-type effect when alcohol is consumed concomitantly. Patients should be specifically advised not to drink. Tinidazole may also be used as a 2 g stat dose. Clindamycin is the other antibiotic that may be used orally or by vaginal application; 2% clindamycin vaginal cream may be applied once a night for 7 nights. Further, 300 mg twice daily is an accepted oral regime. Clindamycin has a more favourable tolerability compared with metronidazole, though patients should be warned of diarrhoea. If this occurs, the drug should be stopped due to the risk of developing antibiotic-related colitis. Due to poorer systemic availability, the gel and cream preparations are better tolerated than the oral regimes.

The two types of non-antimicrobial treatments that have been used to treat BV are acidification and application of lactobacilli. 'Acidification' involves the application of acetic acid gel or lactic acid pessaries to reduce the pH of the vagina. Outcomes were poor when compared with antibiotics and their routine use is therefore not recommended. However, one trial has shown a possible benefit in the prevention of recurrence. Topical or oral treatment with *Lactobacillus* species may have a role to play in the treatment of BV. Further, some small studies have shown a possible benefit in their use. There is no consensus on the dose or the species of *Lactobacillus* required. There is no harm in advising patients to take live yogurts, as long as they are aware that evidence regarding their use is inconclusive.

Recurring BV and its management may represent a challenge, as the necessary duration of treatment needs to be decided. This is partly because BV frequently recurs by 3 months in patients, no matter what treatment regime is used. Weekly vaginal metronidazole has been shown to be effective but is associated with a greater incidence of vaginal candidiasis. In the most resistant cases, a combination of antibiotics, acidification and *Lactobacillus* provision may need to be employed. If the patient has an intrauterine contraceptive device, this should be removed and alternative forms of contraception discussed.

The risks of BV to the fetus in pregnancy and of ascending infection in gynaecological surgery have been mentioned. Therefore, it is recommended that BV be treated in pregnancy and prior to surgery. One should repeat swabs, where possible, 1 month after treatment to confirm whether BV has actually been cleared. Unfortunately, despite the strong link of BV to adverse effects on the pregnancy, metronidazole has not been shown to reduce the incidence of adverse pregnancy outcomes associated with BV. In some cases, it has been shown to increase the risk of preterm birth. Recent studies have suggested a possible reduction in preterm birth rates with the use of clindamycin rather than metronidazole. This, more than anything else, is a demonstration of our lack of full understanding of the aetiopathogenesis of the condition.

Examination practice: use of drugs and toxins in pregnancy

Options for questions 31–33:

a leflunomide

b montelukast

c ramipril

d methyldopa

e prazosin

f warfarin

g labetalol

h metformin

i cyclosporin.

Instructions: The following questions explore the potential problems associated with the use of drugs in pregnancy. Match the description of the side effects with the drug from the list most likely to cause them. Each option may be used once, more than once or not at all.

31 Exposure in latter half of pregnancy may cause reduced blood flow to fetal kidneys and rarely cause fetal renal failure.

32 Exposure in the first trimester is associated with embryopathy consisting of nasal hypoplasia, stippled epiphysis and limb deformities.

33 Has a long half-life, with active metabolites detected up to 2 years after stopping the drug.

34 A woman who is 10 weeks pregnant presents at her first antenatal appointment. She is a current smoker and is keen to give up. Which of the following statements are true?

    a Studies have shown that CBT is effective in helping women who are pregnant to quit smoking.

    b There is strong evidence that nicotine replacement therapy (NRT) results in the newborn child needing special care after birth.

    c Bupropion is first-line treatment for pregnant women with epilepsy who wish to quit smoking.

    d Urine or saliva cotinine tests are more accurate than carbon monoxide (CO) tests in detecting whether the patient has been smoking.

    e Provision of incentives to quit smoking has been shown to be effective in pregnant women in countries other than the UK.

35 Which of the following congenital defects has been associated with the use of carbimazole in pregnancy?

    a Cleft palate.

    b DiGeorge syndrome.

    c Dandy–Walker syndrome.

    d Hypospadias.

    e Aplasia cutis.

References

Abadi S, Einarson A, Koren G. Use of warfarin during pregnancy. *Can Fam Physician*. 2002; **48**: 695–7.

Cooper DS. Antithyroid drugs. *N Engl J Med*. 2005; **352**(9): 905–17.

Donders GGG, Bellen G, Rezeberga D. Aerobic vaginitis in pregnancy. *BJOG*. 2011; **118**(10): 1163–70.

Donders G. Diagnosis and management of bacterial vaginosis and other types of abnormal vaginal bacterial flora: a review. *Obstet Gynecol Surv*. 2010; **65**(7): 462–73.

Kaplan LC. Congenital Dandy Walker malformation associated with first trimester warfarin: a case report and literature review. *Teratology*. 1985; **32**(3): 333–7.

National Institute for Health and Clinical Excellence (NICE). *Quitting Smoking in Pregnancy and Following Childbirth: NICE public health guidance 26*. London: NICE; 2010. <u>guidance.nice.org.uk/PH26</u>

Rubin P, Ramsay M, editors. *Prescribing in Pregnancy*. 4th ed. Oxford: Blackwell Publishing; 2008.

Recurrent miscarriage and preterm birth

Your final patient in clinic is a 32-year-old woman you saw 3 weeks ago. She had presented at 26 weeks' gestation with bleeding from her vagina and contraction pains. You immediately referred her to the labour ward where she delivered prematurely. Unfortunately, the child did not survive and, regrettably, this was a scenario with which she was not unfamiliar. She had presented with similar symptoms in three previous pregnancies. Each ended in miscarriages in the second trimester. All investigations at the hospital had been normal. She comes today distressed about recent events but carrying some papers with her. She tells you she is trying for a pregnancy again and would like to be prescribed Cyclogest® pessaries (progesterone) and human chorionic gonadotrophin (hCG) injections. A friend of hers from California, who suffered similarly, had taken it and it had resulted in a successful term birth. The papers are from some journals, championing progesterone and hCG use in recurrent miscarriages.

Which of the following statements is false?

a Although useful in predicting spontaneous preterm birth, a positive vaginal fibronectin test does not appear to influence the eventual outcome.

b Progesterone plays an important role in the successful implantation and maintenance of the subsequent pregnancy due to its anti-inflammatory action.

c Smoking cessation should be recommended to women with recurrent preterm birth.

d There is strong evidence to support the use of hCG supplementation in early pregnancy to prevent recurrent miscarriage.

e Uterine anatomy should be assessed in all women with recurrent first trimester miscarriages.

Answer: d

This is a very difficult case to handle as poor consulting skills could result in a total breakdown of communication between the doctor and the patient. It is not an uncommon situation where we may be asked to prescribe something about which we have little knowledge. Conversely, we may be confident in prescribing the drug, but may not agree with the need for it to be prescribed. In the setting of recurrent miscarriage, it is important to be sensitive of the trauma that the patient has experienced. It is of the utmost importance to build a rapport with the patient before discussing the evidence for various treatments. The majority of the treatments shortly to be suggested will be initiated by a specialist. However, primary care physicians are likely to be consulted about them first, as they are likely to be asked to refer patients for consideration of these treatments. It is therefore important that one is aware of the treatments available and the evidence for their use so that appropriate advice may be given.

Preterm birth is defined as birth occurring before 37 weeks' gestation. Babies born prior to 34 weeks' gestation experience the highest mortality and morbidity. Loss of pregnancy occurring between conception and prior to 24 weeks' gestation is defined as miscarriage. Most women in the described scenario will have been investigated in a specialist miscarriage clinic prior to presenting to primary care. It is important that we ensure that the patient has been investigated for antiphospholipid syndrome, inherited thrombophilias and anatomical uterine abnormalities. In the case discussed, the products of conception should be subject to cytogenetic analysis. If this suggests an unbalanced structural chromosomal abnormality, then blood karyotyping of both partners should be performed. If an abnormal parental karyotype is found, the couple should be referred to a specialist clinical geneticist to discuss their options. Screening for diabetes, thyroid disease and antithyroid antibodies should also be performed as they have been linked with recurrent miscarriage. Vaginal swabs to rule out BV and other abnormal vaginal flora should also be performed. In the presence of BV, treatment with clindamycin early in the second trimester may reduce the risk of miscarriage.

Aspirin and unfractionated heparin used in combination have been shown to significantly increase the chance of a live birth in women who have antiphospholipid syndrome. However, the latter does increase the risk of heparin-induced thrombocytopenia. Therefore, low-molecular weight heparin (e.g. Enoxaparin 40 mg daily, delivered subcutaneously) may be preferred in pregnancy. Platelets should be monitored nonetheless. Patients on this regime should be closely monitored in the antenatal period. This monitoring is usually carried out in specialist obstetric clinics. Use of corticosteroids and intravenous Ig is not recommended in antiphospholipid syndrome, as their use may be associated with greater harm. Heparin therapy is also used in thrombophilia-associated miscarriage. Aspirin and heparin combinations are also used by specialists when no cause for recurrent miscarriage is found. Evidence for their use in this context is not strong.

Cervical cerclage for an 'incompetent cervix' has been used as a technique to reduce the possibility of preterm birth for over 100 years. It involves placing a suture in the cervix to offer it mechanical and structural support. In the presence of a history of previous mid-trimester loss or preterm birth, cerclage is offered to women if the cervix is found to be shorter than 25 mm on ultrasound surveillance of cervical length. This should be offered prior to 24 weeks' gestation and in singleton pregnancies. Cerclage in multiple pregnancies is associated with an increased risk of preterm birth and is, therefore, not recommended.

Progesterone is known to be important for successful implantation and subsequent maintenance of pregnancy. This raises the possibility of supplementing the pregnancy with progesterone to reduce the rate of spontaneous miscarriage and preterm birth. However, evidence for its use is inconclusive. At present, the Progesterone in Recurrent Miscarriage (PROMISE) trial, a large multi-centre study, is looking at the use of first-trimester progesterone in women with unexplained miscarriages. Despite the lack of conclusive evidence, many obstetricians encourage its use. Intramuscular progesterone given weekly between 16 and 36 weeks is encouraged by some (Iams and Berghella). Some specialists also use vaginal progesterone (e.g. Cyclogest® pessaries 400 mg twice per day).

Due to the link between PCOS and miscarriage, the use of metformin has been suggested for use in preventing miscarriage. This is because it improves sensitivity to insulin, resistance to which is believed to be the reason for an increased miscarriage rate. Although uncontrolled studies suggest it may be beneficial in pregnancy, evidence from RCTs for its use remains unconvincing. Similarly, pituitary suppression prior to pregnancy to prevent luteinising hormone (LH) hypersecretion (which may be present in PCOS) is also not recommended.

The use of hCG is not supported by evidence. An international double-blind placebo-controlled trial compared hCG with placebo in the management of recurrent abortion. Placebo or hCG was given up to week 16 of the pregnancy. Of the 75 patients who completed the trial, 36 received hCG and 39 received placebo. Successful pregnancy rates were 83% versus 79% ($P = 0.45$). Although a multivitamin preparation for pregnancy is recommended, there is no evidence that vitamin C and E specifically reduce the rate of preterm birth.

Examination practice: complications of the peripartum period

Options for questions 36–38:

a   atosiban

b   labetalol

c   methyldopa

d   ramipril

e   ergometrine

f   ursodeoxycholic acid

g   intravenous acyclovir and caesarean section

h   zidovudine infusion

i   anti-D Ig

j   none of the above.

Instructions: Each of the following clinical scenarios relate to women presenting to you in labour. For each scenario, select the single most appropriate treatment from the list of options provided. Each option may be used once, more than once or not at all.

36   A 29-year-old asthmatic woman presents at 39 weeks pregnant. She complains of a mild headache. Her blood pressure (BP) has been measured at 180/110 mmHg on two separate occasions and she has 2+ proteinuria.

37   A woman 28 weeks pregnant presents with regular tightenings. Preterm labour is diagnosed. It is deemed useful to delay labour to organise in utero transfer to a specialist centre.

38   A 28-year-old woman presents in established labour. On examination, cord prolapse is found.

39   You are the on-call obstetric senior house officer. The midwife calls you to the labour ward to deal with an irate husband. He is demanding an emergency caesarean section for his wife who has a breech presentation but is not in active labour. Which of the following is not an indication for a category 1 caesarean section?

a Placental abruption with a cardiotocography (CTG) recording showing fetal bradycardia.

b Rupture of previous caesarean scar.

c Visible cord prolapse.

d Primary genital herpes in the third trimester.

e Scalp pH of <7.20.

40 Regarding neonatal resuscitation, which of the following statements is false?

a Due to a prominent occiput, the prone position in the neonate results in a flexed head posture that compromises the airway.

b If baby is not breathing adequately by 90 seconds, give three 'inflation breaths'.

c The compression : ventilation ratio is 3 : 1.

d If drugs such as adrenaline are used, then they are best delivered close to the heart, usually via an umbilical venous catheter.

e In the rare case of large-volume blood loss, isotonic crystalloid is preferred over albumin for emergency volume replacement.

References

Collins S, Arulkumaran S, Hayes K, et al., editors. Oxford Handbook of Obstetrics and Gynaecology. 2nd ed. Oxford: Oxford University Press; 2008.

Harrison RF. Human chorionic gonadotrophin (hCG) in the management of recurrent abortion; results of a multi-centre placebo-controlled study. Eur J Obstet Gynecol Reprod Biol. 1992; 47(3): 175–9.

Iams JD, Berghella V. Care for women with prior pre term birth. Am J Obstet Gynecol. 2010; 203(2): 89–100.

NICE. Hypertension in Pregnancy: NICE clinical guidelines CG 107. London: NICE; 2010. www.nice.org.uk/cg107

Resuscitation Council (UK). Newborn life support. Resuscitation Guidelines 2010. London: Resuscitation Council (UK); 2010. pp. 118–27. Available at: www.resus.org.uk/pages/nls.pdf (accessed 10 December 2010).

RGOG. Cervical Cerclage. Green-top Guideline No. 60. London: Guidelines and

Audit Committee of the RCOG; May 2011. Available at: www.rcog.org.uk/files/rcog-corp/GTG60cervicalcerclage.pdf (accessed 7 March 2012).

RGOG. *The Investigation and Treatment of Couples with Recurrent First-Trimester and Second-Trimester Miscarriage*. Green-top Guideline No. 17. London: Guidelines and Audit Committee of the RCOG; April 2011. Available at: www.rcog.org.uk/files/rcog-corp/GTG17recurrentmiscarriage.pdf (accessed 7 March 2012).

RGOG. *Tocolytic Drugs for Women in Preterm Labour*. Green-top Guideline No. 1B. London: Guidelines and Audit Committee of the RCOG; February 2011. Available at: www.rcog.org.uk/files/rcog-corp/GTG1b26072011.pdf (accessed 7 March 2012).

Pregnancy and malaria

A 30-year-old woman presents to your surgery on Wednesday morning as an emergency appointment. She is 14 weeks into an uncomplicated pregnancy. A look at her notes tells you that she is medically well and on no regular medications. She appears emotional as she sits down. She tells you that she has just received information that her elderly father in Somalia has been taken seriously ill and she is travelling there in the morning to be with him. She is aware that there is a malaria outbreak in her village and was hoping you could give her immunisation against it. She hopes to be back in the UK within a month.

Which of the following statements is true?

a   It is too late to immunise her against malaria as this should be done 2 weeks prior to travel to an endemic area.

b   She should be reassured that no treatment is required, as her risk of contracting malaria is low.

c   Bite prevention is the only treatment available, as chemoprophylactic drugs are contraindicated in the second trimester of pregnancy.

d   Skin repellents such as N,N-Diethyl-*meta*-toluamide (DEET) must be avoided as they are known to be harmful to the fetus.

e   Chloroquine is safe in pregnancy but resistance to it is high.

Although a collapse from a ruptured ectopic pregnancy is not imminent here, the urgent nature of this appointment is wholly justified, as malaria is a life-threatening condition that is wholly preventable. The risks to the mother and fetus are significant. There is a greater risk of maternal death, stillbirth and miscarriage in malaria. In this case, we have a pregnant patient travelling to a highly endemic area in the next 24 hours. In the first instance, the mentioned risks should be relayed to any pregnant woman intending to travel to a high-risk area for malaria. Attempts should be made to dissuade her from travel due to the potential mortality and morbidity from contracting malaria. In this case, it may be difficult to do so, hence, an active management plan will need to be made.

The patient should be informed that there is no vaccine available against malaria and the well-known ABCD approach should be communicated. The Health Protection Agency (HPA) website carries useful information for patients.

A   Awareness of malaria. This is imperative – in having this consultation today, your patient has demonstrated this already. The patient needs to be aware that the risk of contracting malaria in sub-Saharan Africa without chemoprophylaxis can be as high as 1 in 50. The risk of malaria is greater with bites at night. The risk of dengue fever is greater with daytime bites, so all-round vigilance is important.

B   Bite prevention. This involves all methods of avoiding contact with mosquitoes. Solutions of 20%–50% DEET should be applied to the skin; the higher concentration solution is preferred. Studies of 20% solutions have demonstrated no harm to the mother or fetus, despite the presence of DEET in cord blood in some cases. Extensive use of 50% solutions over the years, without any adverse effects, means that it can be recommended with reasonable confidence. Sprays, insecticide-impregnated bed nets, long-sleeved shirts and long pants, appropriate footwear and electrically heated mats used to kill mosquitoes should all be used where possible.

C Chemoprophylaxis. Specialist advice may need to be sought to ensure the most up-to-date advice can be provided to the patient. Telephone advice can be sought from the National Travel Health Network and Centre. Queries can also be faxed to the HPA Malaria Reference Laboratory at the London School of Hygiene and Travel Medicine and non-urgent enquires can be made by filling in a form available on the HPA website. The stated time for replies is 3 days.

Chloroquine and proguanil are known to be safe in pregnancy; however, resistance is high in many areas, hence they are not efficacious. If the antifolate proguanil is used, then the pregnant mother should receive 5 mg of folic acid daily. In chloroquine-resistant areas, the drug of choice is mefloquine. The suggested regime is 250 mg once per week. Since its action is against the red cell stage of the mosquito life cycle, it should be taken continuously for 4 weeks after leaving the endemic area. Ideally, it should be started 2½ weeks prior to leaving for the endemic area, but that is not possible in this scenario. Mefloquine is contraindicated if a history of psychiatric disorders or convulsions is present. If mefloquine cannot be used, then Malarone (atovaquone and proguanil) is an alternative option. There is limited data available on its safety in pregnancy. If used, one tablet daily, started 1–2 days before travelling and continuing for 1 week after return (as it disrupts the development of the replicating parasites in the liver), is the suggested regime. Doxycycline and primaquine are contraindicated in pregnancy.

D Diagnosis and treatment carried out promptly. Patients should be advised that no chemoprophylaxis is 100% effective and they should be aware of the signs and symptoms of malaria. Non-specific flu-like symptoms, such as headache and body aches, accompanied with fever warrant urgent medical review. Other symptoms include diarrhoea, stomach cramps and vomiting. The classic textbook tertian fever, in which paroxysms of fever occur every third day, does not always occur and the fever is generally sporadic during the course of the day. Treatment in the UK is with quinine and clindamycin. High doses of quinine in the first trimester are teratogenic. However, the risks of malaria to the mother and fetus are far greater than the abortive risk of quinine. Patients should be made aware that fever or flu-like illness that occurs up to a year after travel may still indicate malaria, hence medical advice should be sought.

If pre-conceptual advice is sought, then patients should be advised to avoid falling pregnant while on malarial prophylaxis to minimise any risks to the fetus. Antimalarials carry a low risk of teratogenicity and, although conception should preferably be delayed until the drug has been excreted, there is no reason to suggest a termination of pregnancy if inadvertent conception were to occur.

Examination practice: preventing disease

Options for questions 41–43:

a   varicella

b   cholera

c   yellow fever

d   measles

e   tetanus

f   polio

g   meningitis

h   smallpox

i   none of the above.

Instructions: The following questions regard vaccinations in pregnancy. Choose the most appropriate option from those listed. Each option may be used once, more than once or not at all.

41   The vaccine for this is considered completely safe in pregnancy and there is no possibility of harming the fetus.

42 Immunisation against this is no longer recommended due to ineffectiveness.

43 This should be given if delivery in unhygienic circumstances is likely. A total of five doses is likely to give long-term protection.

44 Which of the following statements regarding the varicella vaccine is false?

a Varicella vaccine contains live attenuated virus, hence, should not be offered during pregnancy for safety.

b A previous history of chickenpox infection is 97%–99% predictive of the presence of serum varicella antibodies.

c Exposure to the vaccine in pregnancy is strongly associated with FVS and increased risk of fetal abnormalities.

d Varicella vaccine is licensed for use in the UK.

e The risk of spontaneous miscarriage does not appear to be increased if chickenpox occurs in the first trimester.

45 Which of the following interventions would not reduce the risk of HIV transmission from mother to child in pregnancy?

a Antiretroviral therapy given antenatally and intrapartum to the mother.

b Delivery by caesarean section.

c Avoidance of breastfeeding.

d Artificial rupture of the membranes early in the labour process.

e Antiretroviral therapy to the neonate for the first 4–6 weeks of life.

References

Blencowe H, Lawn J, Vandelaer J, *et al.* Tetanus toxoid immunization to reduce mortality from neonatal tetanus. *Int J Epidemiol.* 2010; **39** Suppl. 1: i102–9.

Bruce-Chwatt LJ. Malaria and pregnancy. *BMJ.* 1983; **286**(6376): 1457–8.

Freedman DO. Malaria prevention in short term travellers. *N Engl J Med.* 2008; **359**(6): 603–12.

Health Protection Agency (HPA). *Malaria.* London: HPA; 2011. Available at: www.hpa.org.uk/Topics/InfectiousDiseases/InfectionsAZ/Malaria/ (accessed 29 October 2011).

Hurley PA. Prescribing for the pregnant traveller. In: Rubin P, Ramsay M, editors. *Prescribing in Pregnancy.* 4th ed. Malden, MA, Oxford, UK, and Victoria, Australia: Blackwell; 2008. pp. 205–15.

RGOG. *Chickenpox in Pregnancy.* Green-top Guideline No. 13. London: Guidelines and Audit Committee of the RCOG; September 2007. Available at: www.rcog. org.uk/files/rcog-corp/uploaded-files/GT13ChickenpoxinPregnancy2007. pdf (accessed 3 March 2012).

RGOG. *Management of HIV in Pregnancy.* Green-top Guideline No. 39. London: Guidelines and Audit Committee of the RCOG; March 2009. Available at: www.rcog.org.uk/files/rcog-corp/uploaded-files/GtG_no_39_HIV_in_pregnancy_June_2010_v2011.pdf (accessed 3 March 2012).

RGOG. *The Prevention of Malaria in Pregnancy.* Green-top Guideline 54A. London: Guidelines and Audit Committee of the RCOG; April 2010. Available at: www.rcog.org.uk/files/rcog-corp/GTG54aPreventionMalariaPregnancy0410.pdf (accessed 10 March 2012).

www.hpa.org.uk/ProductsServices/InfectiousDiseases/LaboratoriesAnd ReferenceFacilities/MalariaReferenceLaboratory/ (accessed 17 April 2012).

www.nathnac.org/ (accessed 17 April 2012).

Managing a rhesus D-negative pregnancy

Your last patient in your fortnightly Saturday morning clinic is a 30-year-old woman. She is gravida 1 para 0 and in the 30th week of her pregnancy. She informs you that she has just returned this morning from a holiday in Spain. While she was in Spain, on Thursday evening, she had a little accident. She fell down some cobbled steps. Although she did not hurt herself badly, later that night she had a sustained episode of fresh vaginal bleeding. The following morning, she saw a doctor who understood very little English and took only a cursory interest in her maternity notes. By then, the bleeding had stopped and a subsequent ultrasound of her abdomen confirmed that all was normal. Since then, there has been no bleeding and she has felt regular fetal movements. She comes to you to ensure nothing else needs doing. You look at her notes and find that she is rhesus D (RhD) negative and received 1500 IU of anti-D Ig at 28 weeks.

Which of the following statements are true?

a   All sensitised RhD-negative women should receive anti-D Ig at 28 and 34 weeks.

b Since this patient has received the full dose of prophylactic anti-D Ig, there is no need to administer further doses.

c The Kleihauer test is used in the UK to measure the extent of fetomaternal haemorrhage.

d Anti-D Ig should be given to all non-sensitised RhD-negative women with a threatened miscarriage after 12 weeks of pregnancy.

e One of the benefits of chorionic villous sampling over amniocentesis is that there is no need for anti-D Ig after the procedure.

f Anti-D Ig should be given to all non-sensitised RhD-negative women who have an ectopic pregnancy.

Answer: c, d and f

Blood from a RhD-positive fetus enters the maternal circulation of a RhD-negative mother. The mother produces anti-D antibodies. In subsequent pregnancies, these antibodies may cross over the placenta, resulting in haemolysis in a RhD positive fetus. The purpose of anti-D prophylaxis with anti-D Ig is to stop the mother producing anti-D antibodies, a process known as 'sensitisation'. Sensitisation may also occur by inadvertent or emergency transfusion of RhD-positive blood products in a RhD-negative woman.

On a lonely Saturday morning, this is a potentially tricky case. In order to simplify matters, the case for giving anti-D Ig for RhD prophylaxis will be discussed in three separate scenarios.

1 Routine antenatal prophylaxis. This is something with which all primary care physicians should be familiar. With strains on resources, a community midwife may not always be around to offer advice. Routine antenatal anti-D prophylaxis (RAADP) should be offered to all RhD-negative women who are non-sensitised. Sensitised patients do not require anti-D Ig, as it is no longer effective, and they should seek specialist advice if pregnant or considering pregnancy (hence, option a is false). For the non-sensitised patient, anti-D Ig can either be given as a single dose of

1500 IU at 28 weeks or as two separate doses of 500 IU at 28 and 34 weeks. Informed consent should be obtained from the patient and she should be informed that sensitisation can occur due to a silent bleed, the majority of which occur after 28 weeks. As a result, receiving Ig at 28 weeks will reduce the risk of sensitisation from such an event. However, she may be carrying a RhD-negative child, in which case RAADP will be received totally unnecessarily. Since this is the case in 40% of RhD-negative mothers, 278 patients will need to be treated to prevent one case of sensitisation by RAADP. Until non-invasive fetal blood typing becomes more prevalent, this will remain an issue. Exciting work is being done in this field at present. For example, fetal blood group is being determined by analysing free fetal DNA in maternal plasma or serum – this work is currently being undertaken in high-risk pregnancies. Anti-D Ig is a blood product, so some women may refuse it on religious grounds or because they have safety concerns. Other reasons a woman may refuse may be that the father is known to be RhD negative (ruling out the possibility of a RhD-positive child), or the mother is definite about not having further children (in which case, there is no issue of a subsequent pregnancy being affected by circulating maternal anti-D antibodies).

2 Prophylaxis following sensitising events. The case discussed here deals with a potentially sensitising event. Other potential sensitising events include spontaneous miscarriage after 12 weeks, ectopic pregnancy, surgical or medical evacuation of the uterus at any gestation, threatened miscarriage after 12 weeks (if gestation is close to 12 weeks and bleeding is heavy or pain is severe, then this would also be considered a sensitising event), abdominal trauma, invasive prenatal diagnostic procedures, ECV and fetal death. One may note that a spontaneous miscarriage prior to 12 weeks is not considered a sensitising event. In all these circumstances, anti-D Ig should be given irrespective of whether RAADP was received. For all events prior to 20 weeks' gestation, 250 IU is given. Sensitisation occurring after 20 weeks requires 500 IU of anti-D Ig. In the latter case, a test should be carried out to estimate the amount of fetomaternal

haemorrhage. In the UK, the preferred test is the Kleihauer test, which estimates the number of fetal cells in maternal blood by detecting fetal haemoglobin, allowing for estimation of the extent of the fetomaternal haemorrhage. If the fetomaternal haemorrhage is >4 mL, then additional anti-D Ig is given. Anti-D Ig is given by intramuscular injection (except in those with bleeding disorders, in which case intravenous or subcutaneous routes are preferable) and should be given as soon as possible within a 72-hour period. If this window is missed, there may still be benefit conferred if given within 10 days.

3   Postnatal prophylaxis. This is more the domain of the hospital obstetrician, as patients will receive their anti-D Ig prior to discharge. In this situation, 500 IU is given, with a further top up if indicated by the Kleihauer test in the case of delivery of a RhD-positive child. In the case of a non-viable pregnancy, where the blood group of the baby cannot be ascertained, anti-D prophylaxis is given regardless.

Examination practice: RhD prophylaxis and haemoglobinopathies

Options for questions 46–48:

a   reassure and do nothing

b   admit to obstetric ward as an emergency

c   perform the Kleihauer test and wait for results before doing anything else

d   give anti-D Ig within 72 hours followed by the Kleihauer test

e   give anti-D Ig within 2 weeks

f   give anti-D Ig at 28 and 34 weeks of pregnancy

g   give anti-D Ig at 24 and 32 weeks of pregnancy

h   anti-D Ig is an absolute contraindication

i   refer to a specialist obstetric centre.

Instructions: Each of the following clinical scenarios relate to women presenting antenatally. For each patient, select the single most appropriate management from the list of options provided. Each option may be used once, more than once or not at all.

46 A non-sensitised RhD-negative woman who is 10 weeks pregnant presenting with spontaneous complete miscarriage.

47 A woman 14 weeks pregnant, gravida 1 para 0, found to be RhD negative at routine screening. She has never had a blood transfusion.

48 A non-sensitised RhD-negative woman who is 37 weeks pregnant has ECV for a breech presentation.

49 Which of the following statements regarding the management of sickle cell disease (SCD) in pregnancy are true?
    a SCD is associated with IUGR necessitating serial growth scans every 4 weeks from 24 weeks' gestation.
    b Referral for pre-implantation genetic diagnosis should be considered.
    c In the event of a painful sickle cell crisis, intramuscular pethidine is the opiate of choice due to the low risk of harm to the fetus.
    d SCD is associated with an increased risk of stroke and pulmonary embolism in pregnant women.
    e Vaginal delivery is contraindicated in SCD due to the risk of post-partum haemorrhage necessitating routine caesarean-section planning.

50 A 33-year-old woman presents to you for prenatal counselling. She suffers from SCD. She also suffers from hypertension with proteinuria, for which she takes ramipril. Which of the following should not be offered to this patient?
    a Prophylactic penicillin to reduce the risk of infection from encapsulated bacteria.
    b Folic acid, 5 mg daily, to prevent neural tube defects.
    c Hydroxycarbamide to reduce the incidence of acute painful crises.
    d Pneumococcal vaccine, if not received in last 5 years.
    e Aspirin, 75 mg once daily, from 12 weeks onwards to reduce the risk of pre-eclampsia.

References

Anthony J, Kaye P. *Notes for the DRCOG*. 4th ed. London: Churchill Livingstone; 2001.

Cooper WO, Hernandez-Diaz S, Arbogast PG, *et al*. Major congenital malformations after first-trimester exposure to ACE inhibitors. *N Engl J Med*. 2006; **354**(23): 2443–51.

Moise KJ Jr. Management of rhesus alloimmunization in pregnancy. *Obstet Gynecol*. 2002; **100**(3): 600–11.

RGOG. *Management of Sickle Cell Disease in Pregnancy*. Green-top Guideline No. 61. London: Guidelines and Audit Committee of the RCOG; July 2011. Available at: www.rcog.org.uk/files/rcog-corp/GTG61_26082011.pdf (accessed 10 March 2012).

RGOG. *The Use of Anti-D Immunoglobulin for Rhesus Prophylaxis*. Green-top Guideline No. 22. London: Guidelines and Audit Committee of the RCOG; April 2011. Available at: www.rcog.org.uk/files/rcog-corp/GTG22AntiD.pdf (accessed 10 March 2012).

Rund D, Rachmilewitz E. Beta-thalassemia. *N Engl J Med*. 2005; **353**(11): 1135–46.

Hormone replacement therapy

A 62-year-old woman presents to you in surgery. You note that she has recently been discharged from the anticoagulation clinic 6 months after being first diagnosed with a deep vein thrombosis (DVT). She has now stopped her warfarin. The DVT was attributed to the immobility that resulted after her hip replacement just prior to the diagnosis. There is nothing else of note in her medical history and she is on no regular medication apart from her combined hormone replacement therapy (HRT), which she has been taking for the last 8 years. She tells you that the hospital advised her to stop the HRT. Now that the DVT has been 'cured' she would like to 'go back on it because of how good it was for her heart and bones'. She has also been getting hot flushes again, which she is finding quite prohibitive. She has a strong family history of coronary heart disease (CHD). No family members have suffered from venous thromboembolism (VTE).

Which of the following statements is true?
a   The risk of VTE is increased only with oestrogen-only HRT.

b There is strong evidence that HRT increases the risk of developing CHD, irrespective of age.

c Women who undergo the menopause should be reassured that they cannot fall pregnant on standard HRT preparations.

d Combined HRT protects against ovarian cancer.

e Transdermal oestrogen preparations may be associated with a reduced risk of VTE.

Answer: e

This case demonstrates how medical information can change over the years and the importance of staying up to date to ensure correct advice is given to patients. HRT has had significant media attention due to some high-profile studies, in particular the Women's Health Initiative (WHI) study. As with other matters, the media can easily blow things out of proportion, which can have huge effects on patient attitudes towards medications. It is not uncommon for women to be reluctant to take HRT, despite quite severe menopausal symptoms, due to the scaremongering in the media. Under these circumstances, it is important for the physician to be armed with the correct and latest information to be able to discuss the pros and cons of the treatment.

In this case, the patient and the doctor will have separate agendas. The patient seems to be concerned with her cardiovascular risk and the prospect of developing osteoporosis. The doctor should be more concerned about the recent thrombotic event and its implications on the suitability of HRT for the patient. It is important to set out the arguments clearly for the patient, so that an informed decision is made.

There is clearly an increased risk of VTE with combined HRT. Oestrogen-only HRT also appears to increase the risk of VTE, but the increase is not as substantial as that of the combined preparations. The risk is higher in those who have been taking combined HRT for <1 year. If other risk factors for VTE are present, for example, obesity, increasing age and history of VTE, then the risk is greater. Stopping HRT seems to reduce the risk of VTE to background risk. Further, the risk of VTE may be dose related, with doses of 0.3 mg not associated with a significant increase of risk. Similarly, oestrogen doses of 1.25 mg or more result in a greater risk of developing VTE when compared with doses of 0.625 mg. Oestrogen delivered transdermally seems to be safer than oral preparations. The history of a DVT in this patient is a contraindication to the use of HRT. If the patient is suffering from severe menopausal symptoms and HRT appears to be the only option, then oestrogen delivered transdermally would be the preferred option. Symptomatic relief with the lowest dose possible should be sought. However, it would be prudent to seek the advice of a specialist in such a case.

The patient's rationale for continuing HRT appears to be the benefit it confers to the bones and the cardiovascular system. The aforementioned WHI study confirmed that HRT reduces the risk of osteoporotic fractures in postmenopausal women. The patients included in the study were healthy women and were on combination HRT. There is some encouraging evidence supporting HRT use beyond the scope of primary prevention. Studies have shown HRT increases bone mineral density (BMD), at least as much as bisphosphonates when used for 2–3 years, allowing it to be considered as a treatment option for osteoporosis. It should be explained to the patient that there are safer options available for her. Due to her recent DVT, alternative means should be sought to reduce her risk of developing osteoporosis. Exercise should be encouraged, as this has been shown to increase BMD. Help should be offered to those who smoke and a diet high in calcium and vitamin D should be recommended. Where dietary intake is insufficient, daily supplementation with 1000 mg of calcium carbonate and 800 IU of vitamin D should be prescribed. Plant-derived phytoestrogens may also have a beneficial effect on BMD. One study has shown that 54 mg of pure genistein, the main phytoestrogen in soy, improved BMD as effectively as HRT.

The effect of HRT on cardiovascular risk is a little controversial. The well-established view (mainly based on observational studies) has been that HRT reduces the risk of developing CHD. The WHI study cast some doubt on this frequently quoted assertion. The trial consisted of two RCTs running in tandem: unopposed oestrogen versus placebo and combination HRT versus placebo. Both RCTs had to be stopped early due to adverse effects in those assigned the active treatment (sparking off the previously alluded to media frenzy). Unopposed oestrogen was associated with an increased risk of stroke (an extra 3 cases per 1000 women after 5 years of use in the 60–69-year-old age group). Combination HRT showed an increased risk of CHD, along with higher rates of breast cancer, pulmonary embolism and stroke. Subsequent subgroup analysis has shown that this increase in CHD risk is not equal across all age groups. The increase in CHD risk seems to be pronounced in women taking HRT in their 70s and those starting HRT more than 10 years after their menopause. The evidence for an increase in CHD risk in the younger population remains contentious. In fact, some studies may suggest a benefit in the younger age group. In our patient in this case, at worst, the CHD effect is likely to be neutral. However, the increased risk of stroke after 5 years of use needs to be communicated to the patient.

The link between HRT and cancer is also worth mentioning, though the patient does not seem to be concerned about it in this case. HRT increases the risk of breast cancer. The risk increases with duration of use and appears to reduce to background risk within 5 years of stopping HRT. Oestrogen-only HRT increases the risk of endometrial cancer, which is reduced significantly by adding progesterone cyclically. Continuous pro-gesterone almost eliminates the additional risk of endometrial cancer, at the expense of an increased risk of breast cancer. This dilemma is avoided in post-hysterectomy patients. There is a very small increase in the risk of ovarian cancer with both types of HRT, whereas the risk of colorectal cancer is reduced. There is a very helpful table in the British National Formulary (BNF) that can be referred to when discussing the pros and cons of HRT, as it simplifies the additional risk in terms of additional cases per 1000 women, which can be easily communicated to the patient.

HRT is extremely effective in treating vasomotor symptoms of the menopause, such as hot flushes and night sweats. If its use is strongly contrain-dicated, then alternatives can be considered. Tibolone, a synthetic steroid hormone, mimics female sex hormones and is effective for the treatment of hot flushes. It does carry the same risks as conventional HRT. Although there is no convincing evidence for it increasing the risk of DVT, it is best avoided in this patient. Clonidine, an antihypertensive, can also be used to treat hot flushes but may not be well tolerated. SSRIs are commonly used for treating hot flushes. Venlafaxine, citalopram, sertraline and fluoxetine have been used for this purpose. Low levels of serotonin are probably associated with poorer thermoregulatory control. Serum serotonin levels are reduced in postmenopausal women and exogenous oestrogen appears to increase their level. It is due to this fact that some HRT specialists advocate oestrogen for the treatment of depression. Evidence for complementary treatments such as soy, red clover, black cohosh and evening primrose oil is too weak to recommend their regular long-term use. *Dong quai*, a herb commonly used in China, potentiates the effect of warfarin as it contains coumarin-like substances.

Examination practice: managing risk

Options for questions 51–53:

a   4%

b   100%

c   20%

d   0.5%–1%

e   Less than 1 in 1 000 000

f   85%

g   1 in 1000

h   10%

i   1 in 280 000.

Instructions: The following questions relate to risk and probabilities. Match the appropriate answer to the questions that follow. Each option may be used once, more than once or not at all.

51   The risk of fetal cancer to the age of 15 years after in utero exposure to computed tomography pulmonary angiogram (CTPA).

52 Down's syndrome detection rate with the integrated test.

53 The rate of miscarriage associated with amniocentesis.

54 Smoking in pregnancy increases the risk of all of the following except:
   a fetal growth restriction
   b delayed onset of labour
   c small decrements in academic performance of offspring continuing into adolescence
   d pelvic pain in pregnancy
   e congenital problems such as cleft palate.

55 Which of the following is not associated with an increased risk of thromboembolic disease?
   a Antithrombin III deficiency.
   b Trousseau's syndrome.
   c Factor VIII deficiency.
   d Protein C deficiency.
   e Antiphospholipid syndrome.

References

Albertazzi P. Alternative medicines and the menopause – do they work? *Br J Sex Med.* 2003; **27**(4): 12–16.

Albertazzi P. Managing menopausal hot flushes – is HRT OTT? *Br J Sex Med.* 2007; **30**(3): 3: 14–15.

Amoils S. Hormone replacement therapy and cardiovascular risk [letter from the editor]. *Clin Evid* (*Online*). 4 June 2007. Available at http://clinicalevidence. bmj.com/downloads/04–06–07.pdf (accessed 10 March 2012).

Biering K, Aagaard Nohr E, Olsen J, *et al.* Smoking and pregnancy-related pelvic pain. *BJOG.* 2010. **117**(8): 1019–26.

Bombeli T, Spahn DR. Updates in perioperative coagulation: physiology and management of thromboembolism and haemorrhage. *Br J Anaesth.* 2004; **93**(2): 275–87.

British Medical Association and the Royal Pharmaceutical Society of Great Britain.

British National Formulary. 61st ed. UK: BMJ Group and Pharmaceutical Press; 2011.

Collins S, Arulkumaran S, Hayes K, *et al.*, editors. *Oxford Handbook of Obstetrics and Gynaecology.* 2nd ed. Oxford: Oxford University Press; 2008.

Cook JV, Kyriou J. Radiation from CT and perfusion scanning in pregnancy. *BMJ.* 2005; **331**(7512): 350.

Kenny T. *Smoking – the facts.* Leeds: Patient.co.uk; 2012. Available at: www. patient.co.uk/health/Smoking-The-Facts.htm (accessed 30 January 2012).

Levine JS, Branch W, Rauch J. The antiphospholipid syndrome. *N Engl J Med.* 2002; **346**(10): 752–63.

RGOG. *Amniocentesis and Chorionic Villus Sampling.* Green-top Guideline No. 8. London: Guidelines and Audit Committee of the RCOG; June 2010. Available at: www.rcog.org.uk/files/rcog-corp/GT8Amniocentesis0111.pdf (accessed 10 March 2012).

RGOG. *Venous Thromboembolism and Hormone Replacement Therapy.* Green-top Guideline No. 19. London: Guidelines and Audit Committee of the RCOG; May 2011. Available at: www.rcog.org.uk/files/rcog-corp/GTG19 VTEHRT310511.pdf (accessed 10 March 2012).

Rossouw JE, Anderson GL, Prentice RL, *et al.* Risks and benefits of estrogen plus progestin in healthy postmenopausal women: principal results from the Women's Health Initiative randomized controlled trial. *JAMA.* 2002; **288**(3): 321–33.

Seeds JW. Diagnostic mid trimester amniocentesis: how safe? *Am J Obstet Gynecol.* 2004; **191**(2): 607–15.

Varki A. Trousseau's syndrome: multiple definitions and multiple mechanisms. *Blood.* 2007; **110**(6): 1723–9.

Wald NJ, Rodeck C, Hackshaw AK, *et al.* First and second trimester antenatal screening for Down's syndrome: the results of the Serum, Urine and Ultrasound Screening Study (SURUSS). *Health Technol Assess.* 2003; **7**(11): 1–77.

Walling M. The myths and risks of HRT. *Br J Sex Med.* 2007; **30**(3): 4–5.

Polycystic ovarian syndrome

A 22-year-old Asian woman presents to your surgery. She had some blood tests earlier in the week. She tells you she spoke to the receptionist who told her the bloods had been seen by the doctor who put a note down saying 'advise appointment with doctor, bloods suggest polycystic ovarian syndrome'. She admits being confused, as only 2 weeks ago she saw your colleague who told her ovaries were normal based on a pelvic USS she had for irregular periods. Looking through her notes, you see that she has been to the surgery on numerous occasions with troublesome acne and facial hair. She has heard of PCOS because her mother was told she suffered from it too. She is keen to get her acne and facial hair sorted, as she is getting married in 6 months.

Which of the following are *not* amongst the diagnostic criteria for PCOS?
a   Twelve or more peripheral follicles on the ovaries.
b   BMI > 30.
c   Oligo- or anovulation.
d   Clinical and/or biochemical signs of hyperandrogenism.
e   A raised LH : follicle stimulating hormone (FSH) ratio.

Answer: b and e

Known also as Stein–Leventhal syndrome, after the first researchers to describe the condition in 1935, PCOS is a condition affecting the reproductive, metabolic and cardiovascular well-being of women. Although polycystic ovaries may be seen in up to 1 in 5 women, the actual syndrome affects about 6%–7% of women in the UK. It is more common amongst women of South Asian origin. It is more common in, though not exclusive to, obese women.

This patient's confusion is not entirely misplaced. The medical profession also seems to be unclear about the precise definition of the condition. In 2003, an expert conference in Rotterdam set out to define PCOS and came up with the following recommendation: presence of at least two of the following three features would constitute a diagnosis of PCOS, provided other conditions causing irregular periods and hyperandrogenism had been ruled out.

- Oligo- or anovulation. This is usually manifested as oligomenorrhoea (fewer than nine periods in a year) or amenorrhoea.
- Clinical (acne, hirsutism, male pattern baldness) or biochemical (raised levels of circulating androgens) evidence of androgen excess.
- Polycystic ovaries on USS.

What is immediately apparent from this definition is that the presence of polycystic ovaries on ultrasound is not necessary for the diagnosis of PCOS. Similarly, the presence of polycystic ovaries on ultrasound does not establish the diagnosis in the absence of other signs and symptoms. This accounts for the quarter of women with normal cycles found to have polycystic ovaries as a coincidental finding on ultrasound. An important point to remember is that a diagnosis of PCOS can only be made when other conditions have been ruled out. These include thyroid disorders, congenital adrenal hyperplasia, hyperprolactinaemia, androgen secreting tumours and Cushing's syndrome. Hence, the recommended screening tests include thyroid function tests (TFTs), serum prolactin and a free androgen index.

It is important that the implications of the condition are discussed with the patient. Each of the consequences of PCOS will now be discussed separately, their possible underlying cause and the various treatments on offer to help the patient.

Although no single underlying aetiological factor is likely to explain all the symptoms and signs of PCOS, there is good evidence that increasing insulin resistance plays a vital role. The resulting increase in insulin production affects the ovaries and the liver separately. In the ovaries, increased insulin (along with higher levels of LH in comparison with FSH) causes thecal hyperplasia resulting in increased thecal androgen production. In the liver, the increasing levels of insulin reduce the levels of sex hormone-binding globulin (SHBG), allowing more testosterone to circulate freely. A large number of the troublesome symptoms of PCOS are caused by the increase in circulating androgens.

Irregularities in the menstrual cycle are a common reason for women with PCOS to consult their doctor. The rise in circulating androgens arrests the development of follicles causing anovulation and disruption of the menstrual cycle. Patients should be encouraged to lose weight, as reduction in weight through changes in lifestyle has been shown to improve ovulatory function in this group. If regular menstruation is desired, then the oral contraceptive pill may be considered. If contraindicated, cyclical progesterone should be used to induce a withdrawal bleed at least every 3–4 months. This is because unopposed oestrogen in the premenopausal woman can lead to endometrial hyperplasia and carcinoma. Since increased levels of insulin and increased weight play an important aetiological role in PCOS, treatments to reduce both are being increasingly used in PCOS. Metformin and thiazolidenediones such as pioglitazone and rosiglitazone are known to reduce insulin resistance. Metformin, in particular, seems to be popular amongst gynaecologists, despite its use being unlicensed in PCOS. It is being used to help induce ovulation, particularly in those seeking fertility. There is some evidence that it improves the chances of ovulation, an effect that is enhanced in combination with the anti-oestrogen drug clomiphene. It may also reduce the risk of miscarriage if taken through pregnancy. Despite the fact that there are no known harmful effects to the growing fetus, metformin is unlicensed for use in pregnancy. Thiazolidenedione use is somewhat limited due to concerns of their effect on pregnancy.

Hirsutism and acne are particularly troublesome cutaneous manifestations of PCOS. Treatment involves reducing the amount of circulating androgens and blocking their action at the target site. The COCP is generally used first-line. The oestrogen component of the pill suppresses LH production and increases the production of SHBG by the liver, thereby reducing the amount of free circulating androgens. The choice of COCP is important, as the progestins vary in their androgenic effects. Drosperinone has anti-androgen activity, hence, can be used as part of the COCP (Yasmin®). Dianette (ethinyloestradiol and the anti-androgen cyprotenone acetate) is also licensed for use in the UK. Since metformin improves insulin sensitivity and reduces circulating androgens, it may also be used to treat acne and hirsutism. However, not only is it unlicensed for this indication, good evidence to support this practice is also lacking. Other licensed treatments for hirsutism include cosmetic measures and topical facial eflornithine. The latter works by inhibiting hair growth and is applied twice daily. Spironolactone at 100–200 mg daily can also be used, though it is unlicensed for this indication. It works by preventing dihydrotestosterone binding to its receptor on the hair follicle.

Women with PCOS are at an increased risk of developing cardiovascular disease. They are also more likely to have impaired glucose tolerance and develop diabetes later in life. Hence, PCOS can be seen as the female version of metabolic syndrome. An interesting term used to describe this association is 'syndrome XX'. Insulin resistance in these women, along with tendency for central adiposity, results in an abnormal increase in free fatty acids, providing the liver substrate for increased triglyceride (TG) production. They also seem to show a higher level of hepatic lipase activity, which increases the conversion of high-density lipoprotein to low-density lipoprotein (LDL). The resultant rise in TGs and LDL increases the risk of cardiovascular disease. It should be borne in mind that conventional cardiovascular risk calculators have not been validated in this group. Hypertension should be treated and a glucose tolerance test should be offered if diabetes is suspected. Obstructive sleep apnoea, an independent risk factor for cardiovascular disease, is also more common in PCOS. If suspected, patients should be referred for nocturnal polysomnography.

Examination practice: ovarian problems

Options for questions 56–58:

a   ovarian torsion

b   dermoid cyst

c   dysgerminoma

d   Sertoli–Leydig cell tumour

e   Meigs' syndrome

f   premature ovarian failure

g   ovarian dysgenesis

h   serous cystadenocarcinoma

i   none of the above.

Instructions: The following questions relate to abnormal ovarian pathology. Choose the most appropriate answer from the list above. Each option may be used once, more than once or not all.

56   A 22-year-old woman presents with amenorrhoea. She complains of hoarseness of voice, troublesome acne and excessive hair. Examination reveals a mass arising from the pelvis and clitoromegaly. USS reveals a unilateral solid ovarian mass.

57   A 70-year-old woman presents with the non-specific symptoms of tiredness, cough, shortness of breath and abdominal swelling over the last 4 weeks. On examination, you find mild ascites and dull percussion note on the right side of the chest with reduced air entry. An USS reveals an ovarian tumour, which is confirmed as a fibroma on histology.

58 A 20-year-old woman presents to the emergency department with severe left-sided abdominal pain, which she has had for the past hour. This is associated with nausea and vomiting. Urinary hCG and dipstick are negative. An USS reveals a swollen enlarged left ovary.

59 Which of the following scoring systems may be used for the evaluation of hirsutism in PCOS?

   a International Federation of Gynaecology and Obstetrics (FIGO) scoring.

   b Wells' score.

   c Risk of Malignancy Index (RMI) 1 score.

   d Ferriman–Gallwey score.

   e Melasma Area and Severity Index (MASI) score.

60 Which of the following statements regarding laparoscopic ovarian surgery (LOS) for PCOS are true?

   a Currently, the most widely used surgical technique for ovarian surgery is bilateral wedge resection.

   b In women who fail to ovulate on clomiphene citrate, LOS results in ovulation in about 80% of patients.

   c LOS is indicated in women who ovulate on clomiphene citrate but fail to fall pregnant.

   d LOS is an effective treatment for acne and hirsutism due to the resulting reduction in circulating androgens following LOS.

   e Follow-up of women with PCOS post-LOS shows a reduced incidence of cardiovascular disease and diabetes.

References

Alam K, Maheshwari V, Rashid S, *et al.* Bilateral Sertoli-Leydig cell tumor of the ovary: a rare case report. *Indian J Pathol Microbiol.* 2009; **52**(1): 97–9.

Amer SAK. Laparoscopic ovarian surgery for polycystic ovarian syndrome. In: Dunlop W, Ledger WL. *Recent Advances in Obstetrics and Gynaecology 24.* London: Royal Society of Medicine Press; 2008. pp. 227–43.

Azziz R, Woods KS, Reyna R, *et al.* The prevalence and features of the polycystic ovary syndrome in an unselected population. *J Clin Endocrinol Metab.* 2004; **89**(6): 2745–9.

Ehrmann AD. Polycystic ovary syndrome. *N Engl J Med.* **352**(12): 1223–36.

Gould EA, Kerr HH. Meigs' syndrome; a report of four cases, one having hemo-hydrothorax. *Ann Surg.* 1956; **143**(6): 740–3.

Hopkinson ZE, Sattar N, Fleming R, *et al.* Polycystic ovarian syndrome: the metabolic syndrome comes to gynaecology. *BMJ.* 1998; **317**(7154): 329–32.

Martin C, Magee K. Ovarian torsion in a 20-year-old patient. *CJEM.* 2006; **8**(2): 126–9.

Martin KA, Chang RJ, Ehrmann DA, *et al.* Evaluation and treatment of hirsutism in premenopausal women: an Endocrine Society clinical practice guideline. *J Clin Endocrinol Metab.* 2008; **93**(4): 1105–20.

RGOG. *Long-Term Consequences of Polycystic Ovary Syndrome.* Green-top Guideline No. 33. London: Guidelines and Audit Committee of the RCOG; January 2007. Available at: www.rcog.org.uk/files/rcog-corp/uploaded-files/GT33_LongTermPCOS.pdf (accessed 10 March 2012).

Tiredness all the time

Your heart sinks at the sight of the next patient on your list, a 33-year-old Pakistani woman who has been in and out of your surgery on numerous occasions. She has seen various colleagues about a multitude of symptoms. She complains of tiredness, non-specific muscle aches and bone pain. She has had a whole host of investigations and has also been seen by the local rheumatologist. The diagnosis of chronic fatigue syndrome has been mentioned. A graded exercise programme with the physiotherapist only yielded minimal benefit. A depression-screening questionnaire was suggestive of depression. However, the patient attributed this to her physical symptoms. Two trials of antidepressants were abandoned due to intolerable side effects. She has tried various analgesics for the pain, all either ineffective or intolerable. As you prepare yourself for a 10-minute compassionate listening exercise, she surprises you by asking whether her vitamin D level has been checked during the course of her investigations. Her beautician had commented on it being a possible cause for her brittle nails. You look through her notes and find that a vitamin D level of 15 nmol/L was reported 2 years ago.

Which of the following statements regarding vitamin D are true?

a Vitamin D deficiency is a recognised cause of muscle aches and bone pain.

b Increased vitamin D intake has been shown to reduce the risk of falls in the elderly.

c Very low levels of vitamin D are associated with an increased risk of colon, prostate and breast cancer.

d Vitamin D deficiency has been linked to an increased incidence of mental health disorders such as schizophrenia and depression.

e Vitamin D supplementation appears to reduce the risk of children developing type I diabetes.

f Pregnant women who are vitamin D deficient are more likely to give birth to children with wheezing illnesses.

g Vitamin D deficiency in pregnant women may be associated with reduced birthweight in the infant.

Answer: All of the statements are true.

Many physicians will admit to caring for patients that fit the description here. Patients presenting regularly with a multitude of symptoms, which are non-resolving, can easily become 'heart-sink patients'. However, it is important to be wary of relevant information getting buried under a mountain of investigations. In this case, a seemingly innocuous omission may have been responsible for many unnecessary investigations and treatments.

With the disappearance of rickets from the medical landscape, vitamin D is now rarely thought of as a cause for medical problems. Increasing light is now being shed on the consequences of vitamin D deficiency, which has shown it to be vital for mental and physical well-being and in the prevention of chronic long-term illnesses. With estimates suggesting that a possible 1 billion people are deficient in vitamin D worldwide, across all age groups, it would not be incorrect to call it 'the silent epidemic'. Vitamin D is of particular importance in women, not only due to the impact it has on their health but also due to its effects in pregnancy and during lactation. The

WHI study showed that women who were vitamin D deficient had a higher risk of colorectal cancer. In addition to increased risk of wheezing and low birthweight, infants born to mothers who were vitamin D deficient late in pregnancy were found to have reduced bone mineral content later in life. Most experts agree that those with levels of vitamin D below 50 nmol/L should be considered deficient.

Vitamin D plays an important role in bone metabolism. In the absence of vitamin D, the gut is unable to effectively absorb dietary calcium and phosphorous. The resultant decrease in calcium levels triggers an increase in parathyroid hormone (PTH) secretion. PTH stimulates osteoclast activity, which dissolves the collagen matrix of bones, thinning them in the process and causing osteoporosis. PTH also increases phosphate loss via urine. Low levels of phosphate and calcium result in defective bone mineralisation leading to osteomalacia. Expansion of the poorly mineralised bone caused by hydration is thought to be the underlying cause of bone pain in vitamin D deficiency. Muscle receptors for vitamin D are thought to play an important part in optimal muscle function, with a deficiency leading to muscle weakness and aches. One study looked at 150 patients presenting themselves to an inner-city primary care centre in Minneapolis with persistent non-specific musculoskeletal pain. Of these patients, 93% were found to be vitamin D deficient. All African American, East African, Hispanic, and American Indian patients in the study were deficient in vitamin D. Although this study does not prove causality, coupled with the effects of vitamin D deficiency on bone and muscle described, it should be considered an important possible cause of non-specific muscular and bone pain.

So how can vitamin D be replaced in our patient and what is the optimal amount? Vitamin D is obtained from sunlight and diet. Oily fish, such as salmon, mackerel, and sardines, and sundried shiitake mushrooms are good dietary sources of vitamin D. Exposure of the arms and legs to the right type of sunlight at the right time of day for 10 minutes can provide up to 3000 IU of vitamin D3. Most tanning beds are also a good source of vitamin D. If all of this is not possible or insufficient, then supplementation is necessary.

Supplementation may be with Vitamin D2 or D3, which differ mainly in the ways they are manufactured. Vitamin D3 (colecalciferol) seems to be more effective than vitamin D2 (ergocalciferol) in maintaining vitamin D levels, thus lower doses of the former can be used. Preparations of vitamin D3 along with calcium are commonly used in those at risk of deficiency and in the management of osteoporosis. At effective dose for maintaining adequate levels is 1000 IU of vitamin D3 daily for adults. Severe deficiencies may be corrected with higher doses such as 50 000 IU of vitamin D2 per week for 8 weeks followed by monthly doses; 100 000 IU of vitamin D3 every 3 months is also an accepted regime. Pregnant or lactating women should take 1000–2000 IU of vitamin D3 per day. Twice this dose for 5 months is known to be safe in this group. Since 50 000 IU of vitamin D3 per day for 5 months has been shown to be safe in adults, unless very high doses are ingested for long periods of time, vitamin D intoxication is unlikely. Similarly, vitamin D intoxication cannot take place through excessive sunlight exposure, as any excess vitamin D produced by this way is destroyed by sunlight.

Examination practice: vitamin and nutrients in pregnancy

Options for questions 61–63:

a vitamin A

b vitamin B

c vitamin C

d vitamin D

e selenium

f copper

g zinc

h iron

i vitamin E.

Instructions: The following questions refer to vitamins and micronutrients and their relation to pregnancy. Pick an answer from options a–i. Each answer may be used once, more than once or not at all.

61 This deficiency has been associated with homocysteinemia and poor pregnancy outcomes.

62 This is teratogenic when taken in high doses (>10 000 IU/day) in early pregnancy.

63 The level of this increases in early pregnancy, which is possibly linked to altered maternal ceruloplasmin levels.

64 The use of folic acid periconceptually is not associated with a reduced risk of which of the following?
   a Neural tube defects.
   b Cardiovascular defects.
   c Paediatric leukaemia.
   d Limb defects.
   e Twin births.

65 Which of the following statements *are* true?
   a Vitamin B6 has been associated with a reduced risk of dental decay in pregnant women.
   b Vitamin C is known to increase the bioavailability of dietary non-haem iron.
   c Zinc supplementation in pregnancy is associated with a reduced birthweight.
   d Vitamin C requirements in women who smoke are reduced due to the vitamin's reduced metabolic turnover.
   e Vitamin D supplementation in pregnancy has been associated with an increased risk of type 1 diabetes in childhood.

References

Allen LH. Multiple micronutrients in pregnancy and lactation: an overview. *Am J Clin Nutr May*. 2005; **81**(5): 1206S–12S.

Holick MF. Vitamin D deficiency. *N Engl J Med*. 2007; **357**(3): 266–81.

Mistry HD, Williams PJ. The importance of antioxidant micronutrients in pregnancy. *Oxid Med Cell Longev*. 2011; **2011**: 841749.

Mulligan ML, Felton SK, Riek AE, *et al*. Implications of vitamin D deficiency in pregnancy and lactation. *Am J Obstet Gynecol*. 2010; **202**(5): 429–30.

Plotnikoff GA, Quigley JM. Prevalence of severe hypovitaminosis D in patients with persistent, nonspecific musculoskeletal pain. *Mayo Clin Proc*. 2003; **78**(12): 1463–70.

RCOG. *Vitamin Supplementation in Pregnancy*. Scientific Advisory Committee Opinion Paper 16. London: Scientific Advisory Committee of the RCOG; August 2009. Available at: www.rcog.org.uk/files/rcog-corp/SACPaper 16VitaminSupplementation.pdf (accessed 10 March 2012).

Rothman KJ, Moore LL, Singer MR, *et al*. Teratogenicity of high vitamin A intake. *N Engl J Med*. 1995; **333**(21): 1369–73.

www.healthystart.nhs.uk/ (accessed 12 March 2012).

Female sexual dysfunction

A 36-year-old woman presents to you. You note that she has no medical history of note. She has three children, all born by normal vaginal delivery. She has been on depot contraception since the birth of the last child 2 years ago. In fact, she has not been to the surgery, other than for her contraceptive injection, for 2 years. After discussing the cold she has been suffering from for the last day, she asks you with some hesitance if there are any medications available to improve sexual desire in women. On further questioning, she tells you that since the birth of her last child, she has had no desire to have sex. She lives with her husband and this lack of desire is having a huge impact on their relationship. Her husband feels that she is no longer attracted to him. She feels this is not the case and just struggles to generate the desire to initiate intimacy. Further probing reveals that she is not particularly aroused during sex and does not think she has ever had an orgasm. Sex, however, is not uncomfortable.

Which of the following statements are true?

a Epidemiological studies suggest that up to 43% of women may suffer from female sexual dysfunction (FSD).

b The aetiology of FSD is well understood, which has allowed for the development of targeted pharmacological therapy.

c   Phosphodiesterase inhibitors such as sildenafil have been shown to be effective in improving reduced desire and arousal in women.

d   Testosterone applied transdermally has been shown to improve sexual desire in postmenopausal women.

e   SSRIs are well established in improving sexual function by increasing genital blood flow.

Answer: a and d

FSD is a poorly understood condition. Huge variations in what is considered normal sexual function make defining FSD all the more difficult. Currently, FSD may be diagnosed if the symptoms are a source of distress to the patient (not the partner). According to the *Diagnostic and Statistical Manual of Mental Disorders*, 4th edition, text revision (DSM-IV-TR) criteria, FSD may consist of problems with desire (hypoactive sexual desire disorder), arousal (female sexual arousal disorder), orgasm (female orgasmic disorder) or a sexual pain disorder (vaginismus and/or dyspareunia). The underlying reasons are usually fairly complex and may represent a combination of physical, psychological, social and environmental factors. The increasing sexualisation of society may also be a factor, as men and women's desire to live up to a contemporary sexual norm, which may have been considered abnormal by earlier societies, is increasing. Coupled with the availability of drugs marketed to improve sexual function, it would be easy to fall into the trap of overlooking the complex causes that may underlie FSD. Indeed, there are many who believe that FSD is a condition 'manufactured' by drug companies to boost sales of some of their most prized drugs. They believe that the oft-quoted figure of 43% of women suffering from FSD is an over-estimation. The initial study by Laumann and colleagues asked women a series of questions regarding their sexual function. A single 'yes' was enough to have them classified as having FSD, criteria considered too loose by its critics. However, other studies have replicated their results, suggesting a prevalence of FSD of approximately 40% in women.

Despite the controversy, in this case we are confronted with a real patient. Since it seems to be distressing her, it is prudent to delve into this in detail. One should check if the FSD is 'situation specific'. Ask whether the sexual difficulties are with a certain partner, certain place or a particular set of circumstances. Psychological markers such as anxiety, a feeling of sexual inadequacy and guilt should be sought. History should try to differentiate between the various problems of desire, arousal and orgasm, though a mixed presentation is not uncommon. Various questionnaires, such as the Brief Index of Sexual Functioning for Women, are available for use. However, they can take up to half an hour to administer. Certain drugs, SSRIs in particular, are associated with FSD. History of alcohol use, smoking and illicit drug use should also be sought. Examination should look for tonicity of pelvic floor muscles, disorders of the peripheral and central nervous system and evidence of vaginal atrophy. Reasonable, but not exhaustive, investigations include hormone profile, including testosterone; fasting blood sugar; thyroid function tests; serum prolactin; FBC; kidney function; and cardiovascular risk profiling.

Treatment of FSD is not simple. This is primarily due to the lack of a single cause. Women should be reassured that conforming to 'normal' sexual functioning is not the desired end point, as the definition of what 'normal' is varies widely. Instead, confidence should be restored and the patient should be encouraged to find what is normal for them. Desire without arousal or vice versa may be what is normal for the patient. Contributing social factors should be addressed and solutions offered where available. If helpful, partners can be consulted together. CBT and sensate focus have been shown to be effective in orgasmic disorders. 'Sensate focus' refers to a series of exercises designed to progress the couple from non-sexual to pleasurable sexual contact. CBT is also beneficial for sexual pain disorders, where it may be used in conjunction with various physiotherapy techniques.

There is a lack of evidence for the beneficial role of pharmacological therapy in the treatment of FSD. Testosterone patches (Intrinsa) releasing 300 µg in 24 hours, applied twice per week may be used in women suffering from hypoactive sexual desire who have undergone a surgically induced menopause and are receiving oestrogen therapy concomitantly. The patch is applied to dry skin below the waistline on the abdomen. Patch sites should be changed regularly and treatment efficacy should be assessed at 6 months. If ineffectual, treatment should be stopped. Women should be advised to look out for signs of virilisation such as deepening of the voice and hirsutism. The long-term safety profile of testosterone in women is not well established. If there is evidence of vaginal atrophy, then short trials of topical oestrogen therapy may be used, though the effect on desire or arousal is not consistent. Clitoral stimulation devices may be used for sexual arousal disorder. They are designed to improve blood flow and cause engorgement of the female genitalia. Phosphodiesterase inhibitors are not proven in the treatment of arousal disorder or other aspects of FSD. Some studies have shown some benefit, particularly case reports. However, RCTs are lacking. Alternatives to SSRIs should be sought if the FSD is drug induced. Mirtazapine seems to be better tolerated in this regard. Some small studies have shown an improvement in desire and orgasm achievement with bupropion.

Effectual treatment in FSD, therefore, revolves around patient education. Making it easier for patients to discuss their concerns is also important. Treatment is likely to be successful if a multidisciplinary approach is adopted.

Examination practice: sexual disorders

Options for questions 66–68:

a   exhibitionistic disorder

b   fetishistic disorder

c   frotteuristic disorder

d   paedophilic disorder

e   sexual masochism disorder

f   sexual sadism disorder

g   transvestic disorder

h   voyeuristic disorder

i   none of the above.

Instructions: The following questions relate to paraphilic disorders recognised by the DSM-IV-TR. Match the correct diagnosis to the following
scenarios.

66 A 40-year-old woman is distressed by her intense sexual urge to peep
    through her neighbours' window to catch a glimpse of them naked or
    removing their clothes.

67 During a routine appointment, a 28-year-old woman admits that
    she has exposed herself to complete strangers in the street on a few
    occasions. She finds this sexually pleasurable and does not seem to be
    bothered by her habit.

68 A 32-year-old woman admits being distressed by recurring sexual
    fantasies of wanting to rub her genitalia against strangers during her
    train commute every day. She has experienced these fantasies for the
    last 18 months but has never acted upon them.

69 A 32-year-old woman presents with her husband. Since the birth of
    their first child 2 years ago, the couple have been unable to have pen-
    etrative sex. She reports difficulty with allowing her husband's penis or
    finger to enter her vagina. She has no difficulty in admitting tampons.
    Which of the following statements regarding vaginismus are false?
    a Vaginismus is a common cause for non-consummation of marriage.
    b The presence of an unsatisfactory sexual relationship is necessary
       for the diagnosis of vaginismus.
    c This patient is suffering from secondary vaginismus, as she is able
       to tolerate vaginal entry with certain objects.
    d Vaginismus may be caused by organic disease.
    e The belief that sex is wrong or shameful is understood to be a factor
       contributing to the development of vaginismus.

70 Which of the following strategies have been tried in the management
    of vaginismus with varying success?
    a Desensitisation with vaginal trainers.
    b Progressive relaxation.

c Sensate focus.

d Biofeedback using electromyography.

e CBT.

References

American Psychiatric Association. *Diagnostic and Statistical Manual of Mental Disorders: DSM-IV-TR.* 4th ed. Text revision. Arlington, VA: American Psychiatric Association; 2004.

American Psychiatric Association. *Proposed Draft Revisions to DSM Disorders and Criteria.* Arlington, VA: American Psychiatric Association; 2012. Available at: www.dsm5.org/proposedrevision/Pages/Default.aspx (accessed 10 March 2012).

Crowley T, Goldmeier D, Hiller J. Diagnosing and managing vaginismus. *BMJ.* 2009; **338**: 225–9.

Foster R, Mears A, Goldmeier D. A literature review and case reports series on the use of phosphodiesterase inhibitors in the treatment of female sexual dysfunction. *Int J STD AIDS.* 2009; **20**(3): 152–7.

Frank J, Mistretta P, Will J. Diagnosis and treatment of female sexual dysfunction. *Am Fam Physician.* 2008; **77**(5): 635–42.

Green P. Defining the difficulty – approaches to the diagnosis of female sexual dysfunction. *Br J Sex Med.* 2003; **27**(1): 5–8.

Moynihan R. The making of a disease: female sexual dysfunction. *BMJ.* 2003; **326**(7379): 45–7.

Nazareth I, Boynton P, King M. Problems with sexual function in people attending London general practitioners: cross sectional study. *BMJ.* 2003; **327**(7412): 423–6.

Stanley E. Vaginismus. *Br Med J (Clin Res Ed).* 1981; **282**(6274): 1435–8.

Hyperemesis gravidarum

A 22-year-old woman sees you in surgery for pregnancy counselling. She has a 2-year-old healthy son. During the first trimester of her pregnancy with him, she suffered severe vomiting for the first 10 weeks. At first, this was managed with oral anti-emetics and fluid therapy at home. Eventually, her situation deteriorated to the point that hospital admission became necessary. She recalls that she was losing an alarming amount of weight in hospital due to the vomiting and it was eventually decided to start her on steroids. This eventually managed to bring the situation under control. However, she remembers being told that the steroids increased the risk of her child developing cleft palate. At the time, she vowed not to get pregnant again but is now wondering if that was a sensible decision. She is keen for another child and wants your opinion regarding this. She is particularly interested in knowing if she can take any measures to prevent a repeat of the problems of the last pregnancy.

Which of the following statements is false?

a   Her risk of developing hyperemesis gravidarum (HG) in the second pregnancy is higher than the background risk of 1/200 pregnancies.

b   Multiple pregnancy is associated with a higher risk of developing HG.

c HG is associated with a transient hypothyroidism, thought to be due to the similarities in molecular structure of thyroid-stimulating hormone (TSH) and hCG.

d Ginger has been shown to be beneficial in reducing nausea and vomiting in early pregnancy.

e Acupuncture may be safely used as an option in the treatment of vomiting in pregnancy.

Answer: c

In the early stages of pregnancy, nausea and vomiting are extremely common, affecting more than half of all pregnancies. HG represents the most extreme form of this condition. In HG, vomiting is persistent, resulting in more than 5% weight loss and ketosis. Electrolyte imbalances are also common. These include low levels of magnesium, phosphate and potassium. Urea and creatinine levels may be raised and liver function tests (LFTs) may be grossly abnormal. However, jaundice is very uncommon. HG is thankfully uncommon, affecting about 0.5%–1% of pregnancies. In the patient discussed, due to a previous episode, the risk may unfortunately be as high as 15%. This is a distressing condition, usually leaving the pregnant woman exhausted and away from family and work. As was the case in her first pregnancy, it can be quite difficult to treat, requiring treatments that may potentially harm the growing fetus. HG is associated with a transient hyperthyroidism. This may be due to thyroid stimulation by hCG, which has molecular similarities to TSH. This hyperthyroidism does not need treating and will normally resolve by the 18th week of the pregnancy. Higher levels of hCG, such as are found in multiple and molar pregnancy, are also associated with HG. The severity of symptoms seems to be related to higher levels of TSH and hCG.

This patient will naturally be concerned about her risk of getting HG again in a future pregnancy. Although the risk of developing HG is greater, being mentally prepared may improve her chances of being able to deal with it.

Our job is to maximise the chances of this. The availability of good family support may reduce the risk of developing HG and also reduce its intensity. Foods that trigger symptoms of nausea and vomiting should be avoided. Although not known to specifically help against developing HG, folic acid supplements should be encouraged pre-fertilisation. If the patient is on iron supplements, consideration should be given to stopping them, as this has been shown to reduce the symptoms of nausea and vomiting early in pregnancy. *Helicobacter pylori* has also been implicated in the development of HG. This should be screened for and treated if indicated. A thyroid function test may be performed to determine the pre-conceptual thyroid status. One study has shown that pre-emptive treatment with anti-emetics, prior to conception, may reduce the risk of developing troublesome symptoms in women who had severe symptoms in a previous pregnancy.

Pharmacologically, antihistamines are usually the first-line anti-emetics used in the treatment of nausea, vomiting and HG. There is good evidence for them being safe in pregnancy and they are the only group of anti-emetics recommended by NICE. Promethazine and prochlorperazine are commonly used. Metoclopramide, a dopamine antagonist, is also an effective choice. The 5-HT$_3$ receptor antagonist ondansetron, commonly prescribed for post-operative and chemotherapy-related nausea and vomiting, has been shown to be useful in severe cases of HG. Studies have also shown that diazepam is effective in treating nausea in pregnancy, but its use remains limited due to concerns regarding its addictive potential. The use of steroids is slightly controversial, though they have been shown to be effective in treating intractable hyperemesis. There are concerns regarding their teratogenic potential, with some studies suggesting a threefold increase in the risk of developing cleft palate. Their use is limited to secondary care. Pyridoxine (vitamin B6) has been shown to be beneficial for pregnancy-induced nausea. One study showed that it caused a significant reduction in nausea compared with placebo when taken at a dose of 30 mg once per day. Although it also reduced vomiting, the difference was not significant. NICE does not recommend pyridoxine. However, it is recommended by both the American and

Canadian guidelines at up to 40 mg daily to help prevent pregnancy-induced nausea. It should be used with an antihistamine and started as soon as the early symptoms develop to prevent their worsening. Ginger has also been shown to be a useful option in HG. A double-blind RCT of 30 women found that 1 g of powdered ginger root (250 mg four times per day) was better than placebo at reducing symptoms of HG. It does not appear to have any significant side effects.

Acupuncture and acupressure are non-pharmacological means women may use to overcome nausea and vomiting in pregnancy. They certainly seem to be safe, a fact reflected in the NICE guidelines, which recommend acupressure along with ginger and antihistamines as the three treatment options for this condition. A study by Neri and colleagues compared acupuncture and acupressure with metoclopramide and vitamin B12 supplementation in 88 women suffering from HG. The effect of pharmacotherapy was immediate, whereas the acupuncture group benefitted most towards the end of the 2-week period. Both methods were effective in reducing vomiting. Acupuncture seemed to have a more favourable effect on daily functioning. Acupressure was applied for 6–8 hours a day, which may represent a limitation in its use. It can certainly be recommended to patients as an alternative to pharmacotherapy.

Examination practice: pregnancy and liver disorders

Options for questions 71–73:

a   HG

b   obstetric cholestasis

c   pre-eclampsia

d   Budd–Chiari syndrome

e   HELLP syndrome

f   Wilson's disease

g   acute fatty liver of pregnancy

h   drug-induced hepatotoxicity

i   none of the above.

Instructions: The following questions relate to pregnant women present-ing with liver disorders in pregnancy. Pick the most suitable diagnosis suggested by the combination of signs, symptoms and investigations from the options shown. Each answer may be used once, more than once or not at all.

71 A woman who is 34 weeks pregnant presents with itching of her palms and soles. There is no visible rash. A blood test reveals a bile acid con-centration of 34 μmol/L (normal <10 μmol/L).

72 A woman who is 16 weeks pregnant presents with generalised fatigue, which started before conception. She reports troublesome pruritus over the last 3 months. Blood tests show elevated aminotransferases and alkaline phosphatase and the presence of anti-mitochondrial antibodies (AMAs).

73 A 40-year-old woman presents in the third trimester of her pregnancy with right upper quadrant and epigastric pain. Her BP is recorded at 120/80 mmHg and she has 3+ proteinuria on urine dipstick. Bloods reveal a reduced haemoglobin level, elevated aspartate aminotrans-ferase at 90 IU/L, raised lactate dehydrogenase at 800 IU/L and low platelet levels at 76×10^9/L.

74 Which of the following statements regarding liver diseases in pregnancy are true?
   a If vomiting persists beyond gestational week 18, gastroscopy should be considered to rule out a mechanical obstruction.
   b The presence of oedema of the hands and feet is necessary for the diagnosis of pre-eclampsia.
   c The Tennessee and Mississippi systems are classification systems used in HELLP syndrome.
   d The incidence of Budd–Chiari syndrome is increased in pregnancy.
   e The Swansea diagnostic criteria are used in the diagnosis of intra-hepatic cholestasis of pregnancy.

75 Pick the one true statement from the options below.

a If needed, hepatitis B virus (HBV) vaccine can be given safely in pregnancy.

b Breastfeeding is the most common mode of HBV transmission worldwide.

c HBV viral load appears to have no effect on the risk of vertical transmission.

d Caesarean section reduces the risk of vertical transmission of HBV.

e The risk of vertical transmission of hepatitis C virus (HCV) is high in HIV-negative mothers.

References

Crosignani A, Battezzati PM, Invernizzi P, *et al.* Clinical features and management of primary biliary cirrhosis. *World J Gastroenterol.* 2008; **14**(21): 3313–27.

Fischer-Rasmussen W, Kjaer SK, Dahl C, *et al.* Ginger treatment of hyperemesis gravidarum. *Eur J Obstet Gynecol Reprod Biol.* 1991; **4**(38): 19–24.

Gadsby R, Barnie-Adshead T. Severe nausea and vomiting of pregnancy: should it be treated with appropriate pharmacotherapy? *The Obstetrician & Gynaecologist.* 2011; **13**(2): 107–11.

Jeanneret M, Dawlatly B. Severe hyperemesis on a background of gastroparesis. *J Obstet Gynaecol.* 2009; **29**(5): 437–8.

Joshi D, James A, Quaglia A, *et al.* Liver disease in pregnancy. *Lancet.* 2010; **375**(9714): 594–605.

Kaplan MM, Gershwin ME. Primary biliary cirrhosis. *N Engl J Med.* 2005; **353**(12): 1261–73.

Neri I, Allais G, Schiapparelli P, *et al.* Acupuncture versus pharmacological approach to reduce Hyperemesis gravidarum discomfort. *Minerva Ginecol.* 2005; **57**(4): 471–5.

RGOG. *Obstetric Cholestasis.* Green-top Guideline No. 43. London: Guidelines and Audit Committee of the RCOG; April 2011. Available at: www.rcog.org.uk/files/rcog-corp/GTG43obstetriccholestasis.pdf (accessed 10 March 2012).

Tamay AG, Kuşçu NK. Hyperemesis gravidarum: current aspect. *J Obstet Gynecol.* 2011; **31**(8): 708–12.

Vutyavanich T, Wongtra-ngan S, Ruangsri R. Pyridoxine for nausea and vomiting of pregnancy: a randomized, double-blind, placebo-controlled trial. *Am J Obstet Gynecol.* 1995; **173**(3 Pt 1): 881–4.

Abortion

A 16-year-old A-level student visits you at your surgery. She has no medical history of note. She normally has regular periods. Alarmed by the fact that her period was delayed by 2 weeks, she performed a pregnancy test. To her horror, it was positive, and this was confirmed on repeating the test this morning. She comes from a religious family and knows that they will be devastated if they find out she has been sexually active and is pregnant. In the privacy of her room last night, she searched for information regarding abortion on the Internet. She realises that it can be done medically or surgically. She has also read about the risk of breast cancer and has some worrying concerns about this, particularly as her grandmother died of breast cancer only last year. Though understandably anxious, she is calm and would like to discuss her options with you.

Which of the following statements is true?
a Since she is under the age of 18 years old, you are obliged to tell her parents as their consent for the abortion is required.
b The family history of breast cancer is of concern due to the increased risk post-abortion.
c The risk of uterine perforation during a surgical abortion is 1 in 50.

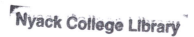

d Paracetamol is highly effective for pain relief post-medical abortion.

e The risk of incomplete abortion is slightly higher if performed medically.

Answer: e

This case presumes that the attending physician is comfortable in discussing and, if appropriate, referring to abortion services. Abortion is understandably an emotive topic and one that often triggers much debate. If the physician is uncomfortable with consulting regarding abortion, they should immediately refer the patient to a colleague who they know would be willing to give unbiased advice to the patient. Under such circumstances, the reasons for referring can be explained to the patient but not used to try to influence the final decision. The autonomy of both the patient and physician should be respected under these circumstances.

In this case, the first issue that needs to be clarified is the age for consent. A person is considered an adult in England and Wales when they are 18 years old (16 in Scotland). Whereas the 'refusal to treatment' of a 16–17-year-old may be challenged, 'consent to treatment' does not require parental consent, provided that the young adult has capacity to agree to the treatment. Capacity is determined by their ability to understand then retain information pertaining to the decision, weigh the pros and cons and communicate a decision. The same criterion for capacity is applied to under 16-year-olds who may be deemed 'Gillick competent'. Gillick competency and Fraser guidelines are references to a landmark court case, which deemed that treatment could be offered to a child without parental consent if the child was mature and understood the nature of consent. If so, they have a right to confidentiality. The physician considers the patient's best interests and the impact on their health if abortion is not offered. The doctor should try to encourage the child to involve either their parent(s) or another responsible adult. Although the Fraser guidelines were initially intended for oral contraception, their use can be extended to abortion. A point to note is that the father of the unintended pregnancy has no legal right to deny or force an abortion; the decision rests solely with the mother and her doctor.

Our patient's intensive online searching has returned some truthful infor-mation. The methods of abortion available to her are medical or surgical. At this early stage of her pregnancy, both are viable options and the pros and cons need to be discussed to help her make the most appropriate decision. Medical abortion involves taking a combination of two drugs. The proges-terone antagonist mifepristone is given first at a dose of 200 mg. This initiates the abortive process. Women are then required to re-attend the clinic to have a prostaglandin analogue 24–48 hours later. This causes the uterine contrac-tions leading to evacuation of the uterus. In the UK, the prostaglandin E analogue misoprostol is used at a dose of 400–800 mcg, depending on the gestation. The dose is repeated if abortion is not induced. It can be given vag-inally, buccally or sublingually according to patient preference. Although the latter two are more convenient, they are associated with slightly higher rates of gastrointestinal side effects. After misoprostol administration, women are normally allowed home to complete the abortion. Pain and bleeding is to be expected and non-steroidal anti-inflammatory drugs (NSAIDs) should be routinely offered if they are not contraindicated. Paracetamol has not shown to be effective for pain related to medical abortion. If NSAIDs cannot be prescribed, then opioid analgesics should be offered. Advice should be given about when to seek emergency help. Compared with the surgical option, medical abortion is associated with more pain, bleeding and a slightly higher risk of requiring a repeat procedure (2%–5%) to complete the evacuation of the uterus. Surgical abortion may be carried out by vacuum aspiration, usu-ally at earlier gestations, or dilatation and evacuation (usually at >14 weeks' gestation). If our patient opted for a surgical abortion, the former method would be used. This method is associated with a low serious-complication rate (<1%) and reduced risk of incomplete uterine evacuation. The cervix may be softened with misoprostol prior to the procedure. This is done by vaginal administration and can be done by the patient. Women should be informed that surgical abortion can be carried out under local or general anaesthetic. Local anaesthetic is associated with shorter hospital stays and reduced risk of cervical injury, haemorrhage and uterine perforation in comparison with surgical abortion carried out under general anaesthetic. Of the women who have a surgical abortion, 1% may require a repeat procedure.

Other post-procedure considerations include the RhD status of the female, the risk of infection and contraception. All RhD-negative, non-sensitised women should receive anti-D IgG within 72 hours of the abortion, medical or surgical. Women are likely to be offered prophylactic doxycycline or azithromycin in addition to metronidazole to protect against *Chlamydia trachomatis* and anaerobic infection. Contraceptive advice should be given prior to the procedure and a plan agreed upon, which may be instituted immediately following. The greater effectiveness of long-acting reversible contraceptives (LARCs) should be discussed with patients. If the patient opts for an intrauterine device, this can be inserted immediately after the abortion. If the patient chooses to delay starting contraception, they should be encouraged to return for review to discuss this further at their earliest convenience.

Many patients worry about the long-term consequences of abortion. Although there does not seem to be an increased risk of ectopic pregnancy or infertility, there is a possibility it may increase the risk of preterm birth. The increased risk of breast cancer with induced abortion has caused much debate in the past. Beral, *et al.* analysed data from 53 studies undertaken in 16 countries and concluded that pregnancies ending spontaneously or by induced abortion did not increase a woman's risk of developing breast cancer. This has been corroborated by many other studies. As the evidence stands, the patient can be reassured that abortion, spontaneous or induced, does not increase the risk of breast cancer. Another concern has been the link between abortion and the future risk of developing mental disorders. Abortion for some women may bring relief, whereas to others it may be a source of regret or grief. Such immediate reactions are understandable and expected. A study by Munk-Olsen, *et al.* looked at national registers and found no increased risk of mental disorders after an induced abortion. However, this study was limited to first-trimester abortions and was based on psychiatric contact in the first year following abortion. As many women suffering from mental health problems may not seek psychiatric help, the study may have underestimated the link between abortion and any long-term mental effects. However, RCOG guidelines do state that patients should be reassured that long-term mental effects are likely to be the same whether they decide to continue with the pregnancy or have an abortion.

Examination practice: contraception

Options for questions 76–78:

a progestogen-only pill (POP)

b termination of pregnancy

c female condoms

d Double Dutch method

e COCP

f female sterilisation

g natural methods

h LARCs

i levonorgestrel 1.5 mg

j copper intrauterine contraceptive device.

Instructions: Each of the clinical scenarios below relate to women presenting to your surgery requesting contraception. For each scenario, select the single most appropriate answer from the list of options provided. Each option may be used once, more than once or not at all.

76 A 20-year-old woman presents at your surgery requesting contraception. You note that she had a DVT 1 year ago. Which of the contraceptives listed carries an absolute contraindication (*UK Medical Eligibility Criteria for Contraceptive Use* [UKMEC] category 4)?

77 A 30-year-old woman presents 6 days after an episode of unprotected sexual intercourse (UPSI). She requests emergency contraception. On further questioning, you find out that she has a regular 28-day cycle

with a 4-day bleed. The episode of UPSI took place on day 3 of her current cycle. Which of the listed contraceptive methods should be suggested to her?

78 An 18-year-old woman comes to you requesting contraception. She tells you that she is at university and has had three sexual partners in the past 2 years. She has never been pregnant and is needle phobic. She is generally fit and well. What is the most appropriate method for her?

79 A 20-year-old woman sees you in clinic. She is concerned about her risk of a DVT since her 40-year-old mother has recently been diagnosed with one. You note in her medication list that she is on Dianette. Which of the following statements is false?
a Dianette is a COCP with anti-androgenic properties.
b Dianette is licensed for use as a COCP but not for the treatment of acne.
c Dianette is associated with a fourfold increase in risk of VTE compared with levonorgestrel containing combined oral contraceptives (COCs).
d Progesterone-only contraceptive is preferable for this woman.
e This patient falls into UKMEC category 3 for COC use.

80 Which of the following statements regarding female sterilisation is correct?
a Tubal occlusion should be performed in the luteal phase of the menstrual cycle.
b Tubal occlusion by diathermy is associated with an increased risk of subsequent ectopic pregnancies.
c Should the need arise, tubal occlusion by diathermy is easier to reverse than tubal occlusion by Filshie® clips.
d If mechanical occlusion is sought, multiple Filshie® clips should be routinely used to ensure adequate occlusion.

e Consent for sterilisation is not required if performed during a routine caesarean section.

References

Beral V, Bull D, Doll R, *et al.* Breast cancer and abortion: collaborative reanalysis of data from 53 epidemiological studies, including 83 000 women with breast cancer from 16 countries. *Lancet.* 2004; **363**(9414):1007–16.

Faculty of Sexual and Reproductive Healthcare of the RCOG. *Emergency Contraception.* Clinical Guidance. London: Faculty of Sexual and Reproductive Healthcare of the RCOG; August 2011 [updated January 2012]. Available at: www.fsrh.org/pdfs/CEUguidanceEmergencyContraception11.pdf (accessed 10 March 2012).

Faculty of Sexual and Reproductive Healthcare. *UK Medical Eligibility Criteria for Contraceptive Use: UKMEC 2009.* London: Faculty of Sexual and Reproductive Healthcare; 2006. Available at: www.fsrh.org/pdfs/UKMEC2009.pdf (accessed 10 March 2012).

Madari S, Varma R, Gupta J. A comparison of the modified Pomeroy tubal ligation and Filshie clips for immediate postpartum sterilisation: a systematic review. *Eur J Contracept Reprod Health Care.* 2011; **16**(5): 341–9.

Munk-Olsen T, Laursen TM, Pedersen CB, *et al.* Induced first-trimester abortion and risk of mental disorder. *N Engl J Med.* 2011; **364**(4): 332–9.

RCOG. *The Care of Women Requesting Induced Abortion.* Evidence-based Clinical Guideline Number 7. London: RGOG Press; November 2011. Available at: www.rcog.org.uk/files/rcog-corp/Abortion%20guideline_web_1.pdf (accessed 10 March 2012).

RCOG. *Male and Female Sterilisation.* Evidence-based Clinical Guideline Number 4. London: RCOG Press; January 2004. Available at: www.rcog.org. uk/files/rcog-corp/uploaded-files/NEBSterilisationFull060607.pdf (accessed 10 March 2012).

RCOG. *Venous Thromboembolism and Hormonal Contraception.* Green-top Guideline No. 40. London: Guidelines and Audit Committee of the RCOG; March 2009. pp. 335–47. Available at: www.rcog.org.uk/files/

rcog-corp/GTG40VenousThromboEmbolism0910.pdf (accessed 10 March 2012).

Templeton A, Grimes DA. A request for abortion. *N Engl J Med*. 2011; **365**(23): 2198–204.

Recurrent *Candida* infection

A 32-year-old woman sees you to discuss her battle with recurring thrush. She has been to the surgery on four separate occasions in the last 6 months complaining of creamy cottage-cheese-like discharge, vulvar itching and dyspareunia. Swabs were taken twice that confirmed the presence of *Candida* species on both occasions. No other organisms were found on microscopy. On the other two occasions, she was treated empirically with topical anti-fungals. Each time, temporary relief was obtained and symptoms recurred a few weeks later. She is married and has had the same sexual partner for the last 10 years. She is on the COCP. She is concerned that she may be doing something wrong and wonders what steps she can take to stop the infection from recurring.

Which of the following statements regarding vulvovaginal *Candida* are incorrect?

a *Candida albicans* is responsible for the majority of vaginal *Candida* infections.

b Isolation of *Candida* from the vagina is always associated with symptomatic disease.

c Recurrent vulvovaginal candidiasis is defined as four or more episodes in 1 year.

d   Poor female hygiene habits are strongly related to cases of recurring vaginal candidiasis.

e   The patient should be informed that recurrent *Candida* infection is a sexually transmitted disease and their partner should be tested, even if asymptomatic.

f   Weekly fluconazole is an effective way of minimising the recurrence of infection.

Answer: b, d and e

Although *Candida* infection of the vagina is very common, affecting three out of four women at least once in their life, recurrent infection is thankfully less common. Five to eight per cent of women are thought to suffer from recurrent vaginal candidiasis, defined as four or more episodes in a year. *C. albicans* is the most frequently isolated yeast strain from the vagina. Other species, found rarely, include *Candida glabrata*, *Candida tropicalis* and *Candida krusei*. *C. glabrata* is of particular interest, as it often causes recurrent vaginal candidiasis. *Candida* is thought to enter the vagina from the perianal area. It is a commensal organism, borne out by the finding that most women will carry *Candida* in their vagina at some point in their lives without symptoms. A full understanding of what changes *Candida* from a commensal to a vaginitis-causing pathogen is still sought, although vaginal anti-*Candida* defence mechanisms are thought to play an important part.

The role of contraceptives in recurrent infection is somewhat controversial, as studies have had contradictory results. Therefore, a reasonable approach would be to stop the oral contraceptive pill in our patient to see if this causes any reduction in the episodes of thrush. Increased carriage of yeast has also been found in women who have intrauterine contraceptive devices or use contraceptive sponges, diaphragms or condoms. Although this does not translate into an increased risk of symptomatic disease, stopping these measures for a time may also be a reasonable approach. The risk of falling pregnant needs to be weighed up against this. The patient should be made aware of the lack of definitive evidence pertaining to this advice, so she may make an informed decision. Interestingly, one study, in which 15 non-diabetic women were followed up for 6 years, the long-acting injectable-progestogen, medroxyprogesterone acetate (Depo-Provera), given at a dose of 150 mg every 12 weeks, prevented episodes of recurrence in some women. If not contraindicated, and contraception is desired, this may be used as a substitute for the other methods of contraception mentioned.

Candida colonisation is also more common in women with diabetes. If the diabetes is well controlled, the risk of developing symptomatic candidiasis does not seem to be increased. However, diabetic patients are more likely to colonise the resistant, recurrent disease-causing *C. glabrata*. A history should be taken from the patient and if symptoms are suggestive, a test to rule out diabetes should be performed. Interestingly, 'sugar binges' have been linked with symptomatic vaginal candidiasis in some non-diabetic women. The patient should be advised to cut down on sugary food to see if this makes any difference to the recurrence rate. In the case of recurring vulvovaginal candidiasis, and a suggestive sexual history, a HIV test should also be carried out. Having been considered an acquired immune deficiency syndrome-defining condition in the past, it is now well known that most women with recurrent disease are HIV negative.

It is frequently observed that use of antibiotics is associated with an increased risk of developing symptomatic vulvovaginal candidiasis. This seems to be the case in women who already have asymptomatic colonisation with *Candida*. It is thought that antibiotics wipe out the *Lactobacillus* population in the vagina. The lack of *Lactobacillus* may contribute to a rise in vaginal pH, making it more prone to infections. However, the fact that some women may lack vaginal *Lactobacillus*, yet maintain a normal vaginal pH, suggests that other mechanisms, such as competition between *Lactobacillus* and yeasts for nutrients, may also be involved here. The role of live yogurts in reducing the risk of recurrence is far from clear. They may be recommended in addition to other treatments, as long as the patient is aware that there is no concrete evidence of their benefit.

Sexual behaviour may also contribute to developing recurrent, symptomatic candidiasis. There is evidence that receptive oro-genital sexual practices are a risk factor for developing symptomatic candidiasis. Increased frequency of sex may also increase the risk of infection. *Candida* carriage is more common in uncircumcised men. Transmission from asymptomatic male partners seems unlikely. Poor female hygiene does not seem to be related to candidiasis. The patient should be advised to wear loose clothing and cotton underwear to allow plentiful ventilation, though the benefit of this seems unclear. Local allergens or hypersensitivity reactions – for example, to piercings – may also damage vaginal defence mechanisms and contribute to an increased risk of transmission and infection. If suspected, they should be removed if possible.

Other factors that play a role in symptomatic disease, which may not be applicable to our patient, are pregnancy and genetics. Higher levels of oestrogens are thought to enhance the adherence of *Candida* to the epithelial lining of the vagina (the same mechanism may also be involved in increased infections with oral contraceptives). A strong family history may suggest a genetic susceptibility to disease.

Acute infection may vary in its presentation, but symptoms include little or copious discharge, usually described as cottage cheese like, pruritus, dyspareunia and vaginal soreness. Examination may reveal the typical discharge and erythema as well as swelling of the female genitalia. Despite the availability and frequent use of over the counter treatments, several studies have shown that patient self-diagnosis is generally unreliable, resulting in an overuse of treatment. The lack of a simple diagnostic test means that diagnosis is based on clinical presentation, microscopy with or without culture and pH testing.

Acute infection responds well to topical or oral azoles. Topical azoles are available over the counter and are generally very effective and well tolerated. Single-dose therapy (e.g. vaginal pessary clotrimazole 500 mg, oral fluconazole 150 mg) is also effective and may be more acceptable to patients. Recurrent disease is more difficult to treat. Mycological culture should be obtained to identify the *Candida* species responsible for the infection. *Candida* species resistant to azoles are thankfully rare. In recurrent disease, topical or oral azole therapy should be started and continued until the patient is symptom free. A repeat culture should be performed to confirm that infection has been cleared. Half of women will relapse if a maintenance regime is not started. Acceptable maintenance regimes include weekly 500 mg clotrimazole pessaries or 150 mg fluconazole, or a daily regime of 100 mg ketoconazole. The latter has a poorer safety profile, hence is rarely used. Unfortunately, a symptomatic relapse is seen in 50% of women within a short time of stopping treatment. A long-term cure, therefore, remains elusive. The usual method is to repeat 6-monthly suppressive regimes. *C. glabrata* has a higher resistance to azole therapy, making its treatment particularly difficult. Vaginal boric acid (600 mg in a gelatine capsule), amphotericin B suppositories and topical flucytosine have shown some beneficial effect.

Examination practice: diseases of the female genitalia

Options for questions 81–83:

a candidiasis

b BV

c herpes simplex

d trichomoniasis

e contact dermatitis

f lichen planus

g human papillomavirus (HPV)

h foreign body

i atrophic vaginitis.

Instructions: The following questions refer to women presenting with vulvo-vaginitis. Pick the most likely cause for each scenario from the listed options. Each option may be used once, more than once or not at all.

81 A 48-year-old woman presents with chronic vulvovaginitis. Examination reveals a sore-looking labia and introitus. Some white streaks in a

fern-like pattern are seen. Mucosal biopsy reveals band-like infiltrate of lymphocytes at the junction of the dermis and epidermis.

82 A 22-year-old woman presents with a 1-week history of increased yellow frothy vaginal discharge, pruritus and dysuria. Examination of the discharge reveals a pH of 5.0 and presence of mobile microorganisms. She has had three different sexual partners in the last month.

83 A 60-year-old postmenopausal woman complains of vaginal dryness, dysuria, post-coital bleeding and dyspareunia. Examination reveals a thin erythematous mucosa with a narrow introitus.

84 Consider these statements regarding genital warts. Which are *not* true?
   a The majority of visible genital warts are caused by HPV types 6 and 11.
   b Cervarix®, a vaccine used in the UK, protects against HPV types 6, 11, 16 and 18.
   c Podophyllotoxin and imiquimod cream are licensed for the treatment of anogenital warts in non-pregnant women.
   d Cryotherapy is contraindicated in the treatment of genital warts, as it may cause extensive spreading of lesions.
   e Latent HPV infection may become active in pregnancy, causing extensive lesions.

85 Which of the following do not reduce the risk of acquisition of primary genital herpes during pregnancy?
   a Prophylactic topical acyclovir applied from 20 weeks onwards.
   b Avoiding penetrative sex.
   c Using condoms.
   d Abstaining from any sexual contact.
   e Avoiding oro-genital contact.

References

Bachmann GA, Nevadunsky NS. Diagnosis and treatment of atrophic vaginitis. *Am Fam Physician*. 2000; **61**(10): 3090–6.

Corey L, Wald A. Maternal and neonatal herpes simplex virus infections. *N Engl J Med*. 2009; **361**: 1376–85.

Dennerstein GJ. Depo-Provera in the treatment of recurrent vulvovaginal candidiasis. *J Reprod Med*. 1986; **31**(9): 801–3.

Eckert LO. Acute vulvovaginitis. *N Engl J Med*. 2006; **355**(12): 1244–52.

Fischer G, Bradford J. Persistent vaginitis. *BMJ*. 2011; **343**: d7314.

Katta R. Lichen planus. *Am Fam Physician*. 2000; **61**(11): 3319–24, 3327–8.

Linhares IM, Summers PR, Larsen B, *et al.* Contemporary perspectives on vaginal pH and lactobacilli. *Am J Obstet Gynecol*. 2011; **204**(2): 120.e1–5.

O'Mahony C, Stedman N. What is new in the treatment of genital warts? *Br J Sex Med*. 2009; **32**(2): 13–15.

Sobel JD. Vulvovaginal candidosis. *Lancet*. 2007; **369**(9577): 1961–71.

Sobel JD, Wiesenfeld HC, Martens M, *et al.* Maintenance fluconazole therapy for recurrent vulvovaginal candidiasis. *N Engl J Med*. 2004; **351**(9): 876–83.

Endometriosis and fertility

During a well-earned coffee break, one of the receptionists at your surgery approaches you for some advice regarding her 24-year-old daughter. She had had a long history of pelvic pain and painful periods over the last 10 years. Recently, when eventually referred to a gynaecologist, a provisional diagnosis of endometriosis was made based on the history. The gynaecologist is keen to perform a laparoscopy, but her daughter is terrified by the idea of an operation. Her mother is wondering whether there are other ways of telling whether she has the condition. Although at the moment pain is the main issue, she is also concerned about how this may affect her daughter's chances of having a child, as she and her partner were thinking of trying for a baby next year.

Which of the following advice given to this worried mother would be correct?

a   Her daughter should look into assisted reproductive techniques (ARTs), as she is very unlikely to conceive naturally.

b   She should ask the gynaecologist to perform an MRI scan, as this is the gold standard for diagnosing endometriosis.

c Her daughter should have her serum Ca-125 level checked, as a positive result will confirm endometriosis.

d Some women find a combination of NSAIDs and complementary therapies sufficient for the management of their pain.

e The diagnosis of endometriosis is likely to be incorrect due to the duration of her daughter's symptoms.

Answer: d

Endometriosis is a fascinating condition and is a major cause of infertility and pelvic pain. It may be the underlying cause of pelvic pain in 50% of women. Similarly, it affects up to 50% of women with infertility. It is characterised by the presence of endometrial tissue outside the uterus. This 'ectopic' endometrial tissue may be found on the pelvic peritoneum, the ovaries and the rectovaginal septum, a layer of fascia separating the anorectum from the vagina. In rare cases, the endometrial tissue may be found in distant places such as the diaphragm, pleura and pericardium. The underlying mechanism thought to be responsible for this is retrograde menstruation. This results in intraperitoneal spilling of endometrial cells through the fallopian tubes. Since most women have retrograde menstruation but do not develop endometriosis, other important factors are also likely to be important. It is thought that local peritoneal inflammatory factors, which promote the adherence of endometrial tissue in the peritoneum, may be involved. It is also likely that the endometrial cells of endometriosis sufferers have unique adhering and proliferating capacities that make the development of the condition more possible.

The duration of symptoms in our patient is not atypical of endometriosis sufferers. Typically, the duration between onset of pain and surgical diagnosis is 10–12 years. This is because the symptoms of endometriosis are many and can mimic many other conditions such as irritable bowel syndrome and pelvic inflammatory disease. Symptoms include pelvic pain, back pain, dysmenorrhoea, deep dyspareunia and non-specific fatigue and tiredness. The patient may complain of difficulty conceiving as part of the presenting symptoms. The cyclical nature of symptoms, particularly bowel and bladder symptoms, may point towards a diagnosis of endometriosis. Examination findings have a poor sensitivity and specificity but may include focal tenderness (in two-thirds of endometriosis sufferers), palpable pelvic mass or rectovaginal nodules. Ca-125 is commonly raised in pelvic problems. However, it has little part in the diagnosis of endometriosis due to poor sensitivity of 28% in all stages of endometriosis. Sensitivity is better in moderate to severe disease at around 47%. The gold standard for diagnosing endometriosis is by direct visualisation via laparoscopy. This aids in assessing the location and severity of disease. Although staging classifications exist, they are subjective and correlate poorly with the amount of pain the patient may experience and how they may respond to the various therapeutic options. Laparoscopy is a reasonably safe procedure. The risk of a major complication, such as bowel perforation, is determined to be around 1%. Here, the mother should be informed that other diagnostic techniques are available but their usefulness is limited. Transvaginal ultrasound and MRI are available but they are unreliable in detecting superficial endometriosis and adhesions. However, both are effective in detecting ovarian endometriomas. Ultrasound, being cheap and easy to perform, is the preferred choice for detection of ovarian disease.

Management of the condition depends on what is most important for the patient. If pain control is most desirable at present, then medical treatment may be initiated. Most medical treatments are contraceptive, as they work by blocking ovarian function. Since the patient is not keen to conceive at present and wishes to avoid surgery, it would be reasonable to try medical treatment empirically for relief of pain. Treatment is either analgesic or hormonal. Some women prefer to avoid hormonal treatment and manage to get adequate pain relief with NSAIDs, with or without complementary medicine. Since increased production of prostaglandin is a common finding in dysmenorrhoea, NSAIDs, which are cyclo-oxygenase (COX) inhibitors that inhibit prostaglandin production, should theoretically work. However, even though evidence for the effectiveness of NSAIDs is limited, they remain a reasonable option, alone or with other types of analgesics. Hormonal treatment includes COCs (cyclic or continuous), progestins (levonorgestrel intrauterine system or medroxyprogesterone acetate injections) or GnRH agonists such as goserelin. The first two options are commonly used and have been shown to be effective in reducing endometriosis-associated pain. GnRH agonists are usually used second- or third-line in endometriosis management. They work by exhausting the pituitary of endogenous gonadotrophins and inhibiting further synthesis. The resulting disruption of the menstrual cycle induces a hypoestrogenic state, mimicking the menopause. Monthly injections have been shown to be effective in reducing pain when used for 6 months. However, it is associated with significant side effects, such as hot flushes, vaginal dryness and decreased libido. The most serious side effect is the loss in bone mineral density (up to 13% in 6 months) caused by the low-oestrogen state. Therefore, it is recommended to initiate 'add-back therapy' to prevent this loss in bone mineral density. This may be done with a combination of low-dose oestrogen and progesterone or the synthetic oestrogen- and progesterone-mimicking steroid tibolone (at a dose of 2.5 mg daily). Another treatment option is danazol, a gonadotrophin inhibitor, but its use is limited due to its side effects, in particular, its androgenic side effects. Aromatase expression on endometriotic lesions has suggested a possible use of aromatase inhibitors such as letrozole, though further work is needed. The failure of medical therapy means that a surgical approach is indicated, if acceptable to the patient. Surgical techniques are complex and depend on the type and severity of disease and organ involvement. They may involve ablation, excision or drainage techniques or interruption of nerves to disrupt pain pathways. At its most extreme, a hysterectomy with bilateral salpingo-oophorectomy may be performed. Although this relieves pain in the majority of women, it may recur in up to 10% of patients, which is thought to be due to residual ovarian tissue and growth of microscopic disease. Although evidence from RCTs is lacking, some women do find complementary therapies such as homeopathy, reflexology and traditional Chinese medicines helpful.

The management of our patient will be different when she decides that she would like to conceive. Dyspareunia and pelvic pain affect the ability of the couple to have regular intercourse, thereby reducing their chances of conceiving naturally. However, the patient should be reassured that she may not have a problem conceiving naturally, as many women with endometriosis will do just that. The hormonal treatments discussed have not been shown to improve the chances of spontaneous pregnancy. Therefore, they should not be used as a treatment for infertility. Whether surgery improves the chances of spontaneous conception is complex and depends on the type of endometriosis present. Gynaecologists will generally offer surgery for endometriosis in the hope of improving chances of conception. Ablation of endometriotic lesions and adhesiolysis in mild disease may improve chances of spontaneous conception. Laparoscopic cystectomy for ovarian endometriomas and tubal flushing are other techniques that may improve chances of spontaneous conception. It would be prudent to rule out male-factor infertility at an early stage, as this would render most surgical treatments to improve female fertility useless. According to some researchers, tests for ovarian reserve should be carried out on the female also and, if found to be low, then ART should be started at an early stage. Techniques for measuring ovarian reserve include day 3 FSH-level measurement, antral follicle count by ultrasound and measurement of anti-Müllerian hormone levels. If ART is opted for, then surgery may still be needed, for instance, if there is a large (>4 cm in diameter) endometrioma. Ovarian suppression with GnRH analogues prior to ART has also been shown to improve pregnancy rates.

Examination practice: cancer

Options for questions 86–88:

a   endometrial carcinoma

b   choriocarcinoma

c   vaginal clear-cell adenocarcinoma

d   ovarian fibroma

e   dermoid cyst

f   Sertoli–Leydig cell tumour

g   Meigs' syndrome

h   vulval squamous cell carcinoma.

Instructions: The following questions explore women presenting with gynaecological tumours. Match each scenario with the most likely diagnosis from the options listed. Each option may be used once, more than once or not at all.

86   A 38-year-old woman with a personal and strong family history of colorectal cancer develops abnormal menstrual bleeding.

87   A 60-year-old woman with a history of lichen sclerosus develops palpable lymph nodes in the groin.

88   A 38-year-old woman returns for a review at the gynaecological oncology clinic. She was diagnosed with cancer at the age of 19. This was put down to maternal diethylstilbestrol use in the first trimester of pregnancy. Which cancer is she most likely to have initially presented with?

89   Consider the following statements regarding gestational trophoblastic disease (GTD) and mark them as true or false.

    a   Despite being considered premalignant lesions, hydatidiform moles may spread to distant organs.

    b   Serum Ca-125 measurements form the basis of diagnosis, therapeutic response and follow-up of women with GTD.

    c   There are no familial cases of hydatidiform moles, suggesting a non-genetic basis of disease.

d The incidence of choriocarcinoma after a non-molar pregnancy is estimated at around 1 in 1000.

e Surgery is the mainstay of treatment for placental-site trophoblastic tumour, as it is relatively chemo-insensitive.

90 Which of the following investigations would be considered inappropriate during the assessment of gestational trophoblastic neoplasia (GTN)?

a Measurement of pulsatility index of the uterine arteries.

b Chest X-ray.

c Measurement of Breslow thickness.

d MRI of the brain.

e Lumbar puncture.

References

Collins S, Arulkumaran S, Hayes K, *et al.*, editors. *Oxford Handbook of Obstetrics and Gynaecology.* 2nd ed. Oxford: Oxford University Press; 2008.

De Ziegler D, Borghese B, Chapron C. Endometriosis and infertility: pathophysiology and management. *Lancet.* 2010; **376**(9742): 730–8.

D'Hooghe T, Debrock S. Endometriosis, retrograde menstruation and peritoneal inflammation in women and in baboons. *Hum Reprod Update.* 2002; **8**(1): 84–8.

Giudice LC. Endometriosis. *N Engl J Med.* 2010; **362**(25): 2389–98.

Hook J, Seckl M. Management of trophoblastic disease. In: Dunlop W, Ledger WL. *Recent Advances in Obstetrics and Gynaecology 24.* London: Royal Society of Medicine Press; 2008. pp. 135–53.

Hoover RN, Hyer M, Pfeiffer RM, *et al.* Adverse health outcomes in women exposed in utero to diethylstilbestrol. *N Engl J Med.* 2011; **365**(14): 1304–14.

Neill SM, Tatnall FM, Cox NH. Guidelines for the management of lichen sclerosus. *Br J Dermatol.* 2002; **147**(4): 640–9.

RGOG. *The Investigation and Management of Endometriosis.* Green-top Guideline 24. London: Guidelines and Audit Committee of the RCOG; October 2006. Available at: www.rcog.org.uk/files/rcog-corp/GTG2410022011.pdf (accessed 10 March 2012).

To D or not to D-dimer

As the rush finally settles on a Friday afternoon on-call session, the receptionist calls to tell you that an anxious 28-year-old woman would like to discuss her blood results with you. She received a letter from the surgery saying that she needs to urgently come in for review. You ask the receptionist to sit the patient in the waiting room while you look through her notes. She saw your colleague 2 days ago. It is noted that she is 10 weeks pregnant and had a swollen right calf that was mildly tender. Your colleague noted 'DVT possible but unlikely' and organised for a D-dimer blood test to be done. The result came back as 580 ng/mL (the laboratory cut-off for normal is 500 ng/mL). Your colleague tried to contact the patient by phone, but having failed to reach her, wrote an urgent letter stating that her blood test was positive and she should make an urgent appointment. As you call the patient in, she asks you in a state of panic whether she has a clot.

Mark the following statements as either true or false.
a With low suspicion of disease, D-dimer was a useful test in this case to help rule out a DVT.
b The patient should be reassured that the test is only marginally positive, so her swollen, painful calf is likely to be due to pregnancy.

c Wells' score, commonly used for assessing the clinical probability of a DVT or pulmonary thromboembolism, has been validated for use in pregnancy.

d The patient should be referred for a compression duplex ultrasound, as it is the primary test for diagnosing a DVT.

e Anticoagulation, unless strongly contraindicated, should be started in the patient until a DVT can be ruled out.

Answer: a, d and e are true

VTE is up to ten times more common in pregnant women than in non-pregnant women of the same age and remains a leading cause of maternal death in the UK. The reason for this, according to reports of *Confidential Enquiries into Maternal Deaths*, is failure in obtaining a diagnosis and employing appropriate treatment. This may be partly due to the fact that mild leg swelling, tachycardia and dyspnoea are all features of a normal pregnancy. Therefore, diagnosis requires a high level of clinical suspicion. This case aims to consider the various tools available to help rule in or out a diagnosis of VTE, particularly the role of D-dimer testing, as this is readily available in primary care.

Virchow's triad explains the three underlying factors that predispose a patient to an increased risk of developing thrombosis: (1) change in blood flow, (2) change in blood composition and (3) change in the blood vessel wall. Pregnancy is associated with all three of the pathophysiological factors described by Virchow. A detailed assessment needs to be performed to determine the risk of the patient developing VTE. A high proportion of women who died from VTE between 2003 and 2005 were found to have identifiable risk factors. Factors that should be screened for include a history of VTE, gross varicosities, smoking history, obesity, prolonged immobility and dehydration (through gastroenteritis or HG). Known thrombophilias and medical comorbidities such as heart and lung disease also increase the risk of developing VTE. Being over the age of 35 also makes VTE more likely.

Many scoring tools, such as Wells' criteria, are very useful in determining the likelihood of VTE but have not been validated in the pregnant population. For DVT, it involves scoring for the presence of various symptoms (calf swelling >3 cm, entire leg swelling, pitting oedema, tenderness along swollen veins, presence of collateral veins) and risk factors (bedridden >3 days or major surgery <4 weeks ago, active cancer, a previous DVT, paralysis or plaster). A final score then indicates the probability of having a DVT. The D-dimer has long played the role of an exclusionary test for VTE. D-dimers are formed from the breakdown of a thrombus when attacked by the body's fibrinolytic system. A raised D-dimer level may therefore indicate a freshly dissolving thrombus in the venous system. However, the D-dimer is a non-specific test, as its level may be raised in many other situations, most importantly in pregnancy, particularly in the second trimester. Hence, a positive result, when clinical suspicion of a clot is low, will usually mean further investigations are necessary, as will shortly be discussed. If a DVT is suspected then the diagnostic test of choice is a compression duplex ultrasound. This measures the residual vein volume at maximum applied pressure and has a high sensitivity (97%) and specificity (94%) for proximal DVTs. It is non-invasive, usually readily available and acceptable to the patient. An MRI scan may need to be performed if an iliac vein thrombus is suspected. If a pulmonary embolus (PE) is suspected, then the choice is between a ventilation-perfusion lung scan (VQ) and CTPA. The choice of scan will usually depend on the facilities available locally. Patients should be counselled about the association between the VQ scan and a slightly higher risk of the child developing cancer (1 case in 280 000). This is balanced against the slightly higher risk of maternal breast cancer with the CTPA.

To determine the usefulness of tests such as the D-dimer, it is important to understand the concept of pre- and post-test probability and odds. The odds of a disease being present refer to the number of times it occurs divided by the number of times it does not occur. Or, in formulaic terms:

$$\text{odds} = \frac{\text{probability}}{(1 - \text{probability}).}$$

However, the probability of a disease refers to the number of times it occurs divided by the number of times it could occur; or:

$$\text{probability} = \frac{\text{odds}}{(1 + \text{odds})}.$$

Another important statistical concept is that of likelihood ratios (LRs). LRs are a measure of how much a diagnostic test, positive (pos) or negative (neg), will change the odds of disease. They are calculated as follows.

$$\text{LR (pos)} = \frac{\text{sensitivity}}{(1 - \text{specificity})}.$$

$$\text{LR (neg)} = \frac{(1 - \text{sensitivity})}{\text{specificity}}.$$

Bayes' theorem can then be used to determine the post-test odds, from which the post-test probability can be worked out.

Post-test odds = pre-test odds × likelihood ratios.

The usefulness of this concept will hopefully be made clear with a simple example. Our patient has a low risk of developing a DVT according to our colleague who saw this patient previously. This risk was probably determined by the lack of risk factors and an unconvincing clinical presentation. Let us say the risk of her having a DVT is 5% (derived from the Wells' score). She then has a positive D-dimer test. The sensitivity of this assay is 90% and specificity is 50%. So:

pre-test probability = 0.05

pre-test odds = 0.05/(1 − 0.05) = 0.052

LR (pos) = 0.90/(1 − 0.50) = 1.8

post-test odds = 0.052 × 1.8 = 0.0936

post-test probability = 0.0936/(1 + 0.0936) = 0.085.

Therefore, after a positive test, the probability of a DVT in this patient is 8.5%; thus, she has a close to 1 in 10 chance of having a DVT. In view of this and the seriousness of the condition, it would be prudent to investigate further. So was our colleague right to ask for a D-dimer? Had the test been negative, let us see how it would affect the outcome:

pre-test probability = 0.05

pre-test odds = 0.05/(1 − 0.05) = 0.052

LR (neg) = (1 − 0.9)/0.5 = 0.2

post-test odds = 0.052 × 0.2 = 0.010

post-test probability = 0.010/(1 + 0.010) = 0.009.

Had the test been negative, the probability of a PE in this patient would have been 0.9%, effectively ruling a DVT out or making the diagnosis very unlikely at least. This would have saved the patient from potentially more invasive testing and wasting time at the hospital. Studies have shown that fear of diagnostic uncertainty has resulted in an increasing number of people referred for diagnostic imaging. In pregnancy, less than 1 in 10 women are found to have VTE when a clinical suspicion exists. This fact strengthens the case for D-dimer testing when the suspicion of disease is low. However, due to the potential fatal nature of the condition, further investigations are justified where uncertainty exists. Therefore, the purpose of this number crunching is not to boggle the mind but to demonstrate the importance of taking into account the results of investigations in the context of the clinical presentation.

Examination practice: management of medical problems in pregnancy

Options for questions 91–93:

a FBC

b LFT and bile acids

c electrocardiography (ECG)

d arterial blood gas

e D-dimer

f urinalysis

g FBC and LFT

h echocardiogram

i viral serology.

Instructions: Each of the clinical scenarios below relate to women presenting to you at various stages in their pregnancy. For each scenario, select the single most appropriate investigation from the list of options provided. Each option may be used once, more than once or not at all.

91 The midwife refers a woman who is 30 weeks pregnant to you with epigastric pain of a few days' duration. Her BP is 160/95 mmHg and she has 3+ proteinuria.

92 A 34-year-old woman presents in the third trimester with a temperature of 39°C. She complains of pain in her left loin. She has bouts of uncontrollable shakes accompanied with 'the chills'. Her pulse is 120 bpm and her BP is 78/40 mmHg.

93 An Asian woman who is 34 weeks pregnant presents with itching over her trunk and limbs that is worse at night. On examination there is no rash. She also reports anorexia and malaise.

94 Which of the following statements regarding thyrotoxicosis in pregnancy is false?

   a The most common cause is Graves' disease.

   b Radioactive iodine is contraindicated.

c   Carbimazole and propylthiouracil are used, as they do not cross the placenta.

d   The normal range of TFTs varies in each trimester.

e   If left untreated, thyrotoxicosis can be dangerous to the mother and the child.

95 Which of the following statements regarding the management of chronic hypertension are false?

a   Most women with chronic hypertension have a rise in BP towards the end of the first trimester during pregnancy.

b   Angiotensin-converting enzyme (ACE) inhibitors are considered first-line agents in the treatment of hypertension in pregnancy.

c   Methyldopa may cause somnolence in the patient, which may affect compliance with the drug.

d   Chronic hypertension is associated with an increased risk of preterm birth.

e   The use of atenolol during breastfeeding has been associated with lethargy and bradycardia in newborns.

References

Cantwell R, Clutton-Brock T, Cooper G, *et al.* Saving mothers' lives. Reviewing maternal deaths to make motherhood safer: 2006–2008. The eighth report of the confidential enquiries into maternal deaths in the United Kingdom. *BJOG.* 2011; **118** Suppl 1: 1–203.

Collins S, Arulkumaran S, Hayes K, *et al.*, editors. *Oxford Handbook of Obstetrics and Gynaecology.* 2nd ed. Oxford: Oxford University Press; 2008.

Kelly J, Hunt BJ. A Clinical probability assessment and D-dimer measurement should be the initial step in the investigation of suspected venous thrombo-embolism. *Chest.* 2003; **124**(3): 1116–19.

Kelly J, Hunt BJ. The utility of pretest probability assessment in patients with clinically suspected venous thromboembolism. *J Thromb Haemost.* 2003; 1(9): 1888–96.

Marik PE, Plante LA. Venous thromboembolic disease and pregnancy. *N Engl J Med.* 2008; **359**(19): 2025–33.

Matthews S. Imaging pulmonary embolism in pregnancy: what is the most appropriate imaging protocol? *Br J Radiol.* 2006; **79**(941): 441–4.

RGOG. *Reducing the Risk of Thrombosis and Embolism during Pregnancy and the Puerperium.* Green-top Guideline 37A. November 2009. Available at: www.rcog.org.uk/files/rcog-corp/GTG37aReducingRiskThrombosis.pdf (accessed 10 March 2012).

RGOG. *The Acute Management of Thrombosis and Embolism during Pregnancy and the Puerperium.* Green-top Guideline 37B. London: Guidelines and Audit Committee of the RCOG; February 2007. Available at: www.rcog.org.uk/files/rcog-corp/GTG37b_230611.pdf (accessed 10 March 2012).

Seely EW, Ecker J. Chronic hypertension in pregnancy. *N Engl J Med.* 2011; **365**(5): 439–46.

Osteoporosis

A 43-year-old woman visits you for a routine appointment at the surgery. A cursory look at her notes tells you that she has three children, the youngest of whom is 10 years old. She is generally fit and well, takes loratadine for hay fever in the summer and has no allergies. Following the birth of her last child, she was put on the injectable contraceptive medroxyprogesterone acetate (Depo-Provera) and has been on this for 3 years. She recently opted for a 'well-woman check', which was being offered by a private company for a 50% Christmas discount. She brings the report with her, as she has been asked to discuss a few of the results with you. The main result of concern is her dual-energy X-ray absorptiometry (DEXA) scan result. You note this, along with some other relevant results:

DEXA scan result
T-score Z-score
AP spine –0.9–2.0
Left femoral neck –3.0–3.5
Total hip –2.2–2.9

FRAX® WHO Fracture Risk Assessment Tool (FRAX) *10-year fracture risk calculation*

Major osteoporotic fracture 12%

Hip fracture 4.3%

FSH 146.6 iu/L (postmenopausal level 25.8–134.8)

LH 90.7 iu/L (postmenopausal level 7.7–58.5)

Oestrogen 90 pmol/L (postmenopausal level <200)

TSH 2.31 mIU/L (0.3–5.0)

Serum calcium 2.30 mmol/L (2.15–2.55)

Vitamin D 48 nmol/L (50–74)

Weight 60 kg

Height 165 cm

BMI 22

On further questioning, she advises she has never suffered a fracture. She tells you that her periods stopped at the age of 38. She did not find this troublesome, as her mother went through the menopause at the age of 40. She was not keen on HRT due to all the health scares and decided to manage her vasomotor symptoms with complementary therapy, which she found worked well for her on most days. She is a non-smoker, takes regular exercise and drinks alcohol on social occasions.

Which of the following statements are true?

a   The patient should be advised that she is suffering from osteoporosis of the femoral neck, so should increase her dairy and vitamin D intake.

b   Medroxyprogesterone acetate has been associated with a reduction in bone mineral density and osteoporosis.

c   HRT is no longer a suitable option for improving bone mineral density (BMD) in this patient.

d   The 'T-score' is a measure of how many standard deviations the BMD differs from the mean BMD of other subjects of the same age.

e To prevent a future fracture, a bisphosphonate, along with calcium and vitamin D supplements, is indicated in this patient.

f BMD measured at the heel is as accurate and informative as that measured at the hip.

Answer: a and e are true

Osteoporosis is a chronic disease characterised by increased skeletal fragility, low BMD and defective bone microarchitecture. It is a common disease but may go unrecognised for years, as it results in silent bone loss. At the other end of the spectrum, it has the ability to cause debilitating hip and vertebral fractures. The cost of treating hip fractures and the resultant social care is estimated at £1.73 billion per year in the UK. Fifty per cent of women will suffer a fracture after the age of 50. The lifetime risk of having a hip fracture in women is greater than their risk of developing breast cancer. These are astonishing statistics, made more so by the fact that osteoporosis remains under-treated in the UK, despite the availability of effective prophylactic treatment. The menopause accelerates the process of bone loss. Primary ovarian insufficiency results in early acceleration of bone loss, hence increases the risk of osteoporosis later in life.

BMD, a measure of the density of minerals in the bone, such as calcium, is the major criterion used to diagnose osteoporosis. The current method of choice used to measure BMD is an axial DEXA scan, as it is the most validated. As its name suggests, low energy X-rays from two different sources are passed through bone; the denser the bone, the more energy is absorbed and vice versa. The amount of energy absorbed is then used to calculate the average density of the part of the skeleton measured. Results are given as T-scores and Z-scores. They are a measure of the number of standard deviations the patient's BMD differs from the mean peak BMD of young normal subjects of the same gender (T-score) or the mean peak BMD of subjects of the same age (Z-score). Osteoporosis is defined as having a T-score of less than −2.5. T-scores between −1 and −2.5 are classified as osteopenia. Other techniques available include quantitative ultrasound, quantitative CT and peripheral DEXA scanning. The lack of portability, considerable expense and availability of central DEXA scanning has resulted in the development of smaller, more portable, cheaper DEXA scanners, which measure BMD peripherally, such as at the forearm or heel. However, there is usually not a good correlation between peripheral and central BMD measurements. Therefore, the former should not be used to make treatment decisions or for monitoring progress of treatment.

The difficult aspect in treatment is deciding who needs to be treated. One factor that needs to be considered is whether the patient has osteopenia or osteoporosis. Four out of five low-impact fractures will occur in people who do not have osteoporosis. To make matters more confusing, if the cut-off for osteoporosis was set at a T-score of −1.5 and below, 75% of fractures would still occur in people without osteoporosis. Although treatment for osteoporosis will reduce the risk of a fracture by 50%, some women will have fractures despite having treatment. Therefore, decisions should not be based on BMD measurements alone. Other factors that will need modifying and should influence the treatment decision include the risk of falling, previous personal fracture, parental fracture, alcohol intake of >4 U/day, rheumatoid arthritis, current glucocorticoid use, current smoking, premature menopause, low BMI and a sedentary lifestyle. Patients should be screened for conditions that increase the risk of osteoporosis, such as thyroid disease, Cushing's syndrome, primary hyperparathyroidism, malnutrition or malabsorption, cancer and inflammatory disorders. Drugs that increase the risk of osteoporosis include aromatase inhibitors, LH-releasing hormone agonists and anti-epileptics. Some of these risk factors are included in the FRAX details shown, but the clinician should not rely on it alone in making a final decision.

Certain lifestyle advice is beneficial irrespective of whether a pharmacological approach is taken. The patient should be advised to continue with her regular exercise. Low-impact weight-bearing exercise and high-intensity strength training have been shown to increase BMD in both men and women. A diet high in calcium and vitamin D should be recommended. Where insufficient intake through diet is suspected, supplementation should be considered. A diet containing 1200 to 1500 mg of calcium daily should be recommended. A pint of milk with a daily pot of yogurt will give sufficient calcium to avoid the need for supplementation. The benefits of vitamin D on muscle strength and enhancement of calcium absorption have been discussed in Case 13. Calcium and vitamin D supplements have been shown to reduce the risk of hip fractures in nursing home residents. Vitamin D has also been shown to reduce the risk of falls in the elderly, presumably through muscle strengthening. Some studies have shown a modest improvement in BMD with water fluoridation; however, they have failed to show a reduction in fracture rates.

The aim of treatment is to reduce the risk of a fracture. Despite the well-publicised health scares regarding HRT, our patient would be a good candidate for this therapy. Oestrogen has been shown to reduce bone resorption, thus improving BMD. It is likely that the concerns regarding increased risk of cardiovascular disease with HRT will not apply to our patient. This risk seems to be more applicable to older patients who start HRT more than 10 years after the menopause. On the contrary, there may be a cardiovascular benefit conferrable to a young patient taking HRT. The increase in risk of breast cancer and VTE is not likely to be high in our patient either. Early results from the 'Women's Health Initiative', a major 15 year research program looking at the causes of morbidity and mortality in postmenopausal women, that triggered the health scares, looked at patients aged >50 years and found the majority of increased risk in those >60 years old. Women receiving oestrogen (with or without progesterone) were found to have a 33% reduction in the risk of having a hip fracture. If the patient remains opposed to HRT, then bisphosphonates should be considered as first-line treatment. They work by inhibiting osteoclast activity and thus reducing bone resorption. Alendronate, for which there is positive data, can be given at a dose of 10 mg daily or 70 mg weekly, the latter being a more acceptable regime. Other available bisphosphonates include etidronate and risedronate.

The NICE guidance provides, somewhat complicated, algorithms as to when each one should be used. Essentially, alendronate is considered first-line for both primary and secondary prevention of osteoporotic fractures. In some cases, it may be difficult to follow the NICE guidance. For example, secondary prevention in a 65-year-old with a T-score of −2.5, who cannot tolerate alendronate, cannot be switched to risedronate unless her T-score drops to −3.0 or she develops one independent clinical risk factor (parental hip fracture, rheumatoid arthritis or alcohol intake of >4 U/day). If faced with this situation, it may be easier to just switch drugs rather than to encourage the patient to increase their alcohol intake! Bisphosphonates should be taken on an empty stomach with plenty of water. The patient should be advised to stay upright for at least 30 minutes to prevent gastro-oesophageal reflux. Osteonecrosis of the jaw is a rare but serious complication of bisphosphonate use, occurring more frequently with intravenous preparations. More common side effects include heartburn, abdominal distension, headache and muscular aches. If severe oesophageal reactions occur, treatment should be stopped and an alternative sought.

Other treatment options include the selective oestrogen-receptor modulator raloxifene, strontium ranelate and the anabolic agent teriparatide. Raloxifene, the long-term use of which is considered to reduce the risk of breast cancer, has been shown to reduce the risk of vertebral fractures in women with osteoporosis. It should be avoided if there is a history of VTE or undiagnosed uterine bleeding. Strontium ranelate is usually taken at bedtime, avoiding food (particularly calcium-containing food) 2 hours before and after treatment. Teriparatide is a synthetic PTH that stimulates bone formation. It is given as a daily subcutaneous injection and has been shown to reduce the risk of vertebral and non-vertebral fractures.

Two areas of uncertainty worth mentioning are the duration of treatment and treatment of women with T-scores between −1 and −2.5 in the absence of other risk factors. It has been suggested that patients on bisphosphonates should be given a 'drug holiday' after 5 years. This is because atypical fractures have been associated with long-term bisphosphonate use, strengthening the case for a break from treatment. Early repeat DEXA scanning is probably not beneficial or cost-effective and should be reserved for patients who have a fracture whilst on treatment. Women with osteopenia should be counselled regarding the lack of evidence for fracture prevention with treatment and appropriate lifestyle advice should be given.

Examination practice: problems of older age

Options for questions 96–98:

a   calcium and vitamin D supplements only

b   alendronate

c   risedronate

d   strontium ranelate

e   teriparatide

f   denosumab

g   once-yearly zoledronic acid infusion

h   none of the above.

Instructions: The following questions test knowledge of the NICE guidelines in the management of osteoporosis. Choose the most appropriate drug from the options provided. Each option may be used once, more than once or not at all.

96   After a fall while walking in the garden, an 80-year-old woman has a knee X-ray at the local radiology department. No fracture is seen, but the report states that there is evidence of severe osteopenia. The patient is unwilling to travel to the hospital that has a DEXA scanner. She suffers from rheumatoid arthritis and does not drink alcohol. Her BMI is 21 kg/m². Her mother suffered from a hip fracture in her 70s.

97   A 64-year-old sustains a fracture of the left hip. A DEXA scan reveals a T-score of –3.2 at the hip. She is unable to tolerate first-line treatment due to severe and persistent reflux symptoms, despite following the

instructions for how to take the drug appropriately. She has no medical problems, does not drink alcohol, has no family history of osteoporotic fractures and has a BMI of 24 kg/m². She went through the menopause at the age of 53 and took HRT for 3 years.

98 Two years later, the 64-year-old from Question 97 (now 66 years old), taking treatment as recommended, falls again and hurts her right hip. An X-ray confirms a fracture. A repeat DEXA scan reveals a T-score of –4.1.

99 Which of the following drugs is licensed for use in stress urinary incontinence?

  a Duloxetine.

  b Oxybutynin.

  c Doxazosin.

  d Clonidine.

  e Imipramine.

100 Which of the following statements regarding overactive bladder (OAB) syndrome are correct?

  a OAB is idiopathic in most cases.

  b Detrusor overactivity can be diagnosed by taking a comprehensive history from the patient.

  c Anticholinergics, the main pharmacological option in the management of OAB, are contraindicated in patients suffering from myasthenia gravis.

  d Surgery should be considered early in the management of OAB, as there are many safe and effective options.

  e Though unlicensed, intravesical botulinum toxin injections have been shown to be effective in giving short-term relief from symptoms.

References

Abrams P. Describing bladder storage function: overactive bladder syndrome and detrusor overactivity. *Urology*. 2003; **62**(5 Suppl. 2): 28–37, 40–2.

Cardozo L. Systematic review of overactive bladder therapy in females. *Can Urol Assoc J*. 2011; **5**(5 Suppl. 2): S139–42.

Collins S, Arulkumaran S, Hayes K, *et al.*, editors. *Oxford Handbook of Obstetrics and Gynaecology*. 2nd ed. Oxford: Oxford University Press; 2008.

Favus MJ. Bisphosphonates for osteoporosis. *N Engl J Med*. 2010; **363**(21): 2027–35.

Järvinen TLN, Sievänen H, Khan KM, *et al.* Shifting the focus in fracture prevention from osteoporosis to falls. *BMJ*. 2008; **336**(7636): 124–6.

NICE. *Osteoporotic Fractures – denosumab: NICE technology appraisals TA204*. London: NICE; 2010. www.nice.org.uk/guidance/TA204

NICE. *Osteoporosis – primary prevention: NICE technology appraisals TA160*. London: NICE; 2008. www.nice.org.uk/guidance/TA160

NICE. *Osteoporosis – secondary prevention including strontium ranelate: NICE technology appraisals TA161*. London: NICE; 2008. www.nice.org.uk/guidance/TA161

Raisz LG. Screening for osteoporosis. *N Engl J Med*. 2011; **353**(2): 164–71.

Rogers RG. Urinary stress incontinence in women. *N Engl J Med*. 2008; **358**(10): 1029–36.

Rosen CJ. Postmenopausal osteoporosis. *N Engl J Med*. 2005; **353**(6): 595–603.

World Health Organization Collaborating Centre for Metabolic Bone Diseases, University of Sheffield. *FRAX® WHO Fracture Risk Assessment Tool*. Sheffield: World Health Organization Collaborating Centre for Metabolic Bone Diseases, University of Sheffield; n.d. Available at: www.shef.ac.uk/FRAX/tool.jsp (accessed 10 March 2012).

Answers

1 a

There is a theoretical risk of intrauterine viral shedding from maternal herpes zoster infection. Perinatal herpes zoster infection has not been associated with fetal
infection. Reassuringly, herpes zoster infection in the first and second trimesters
has also not been associated with FVS. However, there has been one case in
which a child was found to have FVS when the mother had disseminated herpes
zoster at the end of the first trimester, so the patient should be advised to come
back if any atypical features develop.

2 g

Rubella is a mild self-limiting illness. Contracted in pregnancy, it has the potential
of causing devastating effects in the form of congenital rubella syndrome (CRS).
The risk of this seems to be limited to the first 16 weeks of pregnancy, with no
reported cases of CRS beyond the 16th gestational week. Serological testing
for rubella-specific IgG and IgM antibodies should be carried out. If there is a
history of vaccination and IgG is positive, then the patient is immune and need
not worry. If immune status is unknown, then a positive IgG with a negative
IgM is reassuring. If IgM is positive with a negative IgG or a significant rise in
IgG, then this may represent acute infection and the patient should be urgently

referred to the obstetric team for counselling and possible fetal diagnostic tests. A woman presenting 4 weeks after possible rubella infection represents a diagnostic dilemma, as a positive IgG may represent a recent infection rather than immunity.

3 a

As explained in Answer 2, the risk of CRS to the fetus is almost non-existent when rubella is contracted after the 16th week of pregnancy. However, since there is a risk of fetal growth retardation, all confirmed cases should be routinely referred to an obstetrician for routine growth scans.

4 a, b and e are true

The purpose of VZIG is to modify the course of disease and prevent maternal morbidity. Whether it prevents FVS is unknown. Patients should be reassured that breastfeeding is safe after the vaccine. Possible causes for an increased risk of varicella pneumonia with increasing gestation include increasing suppression of the maternal immune system and increased splinting of the diaphragm as a result of the enlarging uterus.

5 a and d

Measles infection in pregnancy is rare. Studies and case series reviews looking at the effects of the infection on the mother and fetus have involved small numbers of women, making it difficult to draw definitive conclusions. Measles does not seem to be causally related to congenital defects, though the risk of maternal morbidity, fetal loss and premature delivery appears to be higher. When acquired late in pregnancy, there may be an increased risk of SSPE, a rare but deadly disorder affecting the brain. HNIG is recommended in susceptible pregnant women within 6 days of exposure to a confirmed or epidemiologically linked case of measles.

6 e

'Puerperal psychosis' is a term used to describe a range of serious psychotic conditions presenting in the immediate postnatal period, including bipolar affective disorder, severe depression and schizophrenia. Auditory hallucinations, thought withdrawal, insertion, broadcasting and interruption, and delusional perception are all symptoms of schizophrenia. Puerperal psychosis presents rapidly, usually within 2 weeks of delivery. The rate is approximately 1 in 500 births. Women require urgent psychiatric assessment in a specialist unit, ideally a mother and baby unit. Puerperal psychosis is treated according to the diagnosis, with most patients making a full recovery.

7 g

Around 50% of women experience a brief period of emotional instability after giving birth. Baby blues, which may be due to a hormonal imbalance, usually starts around day 3 and resolves spontaneously within 10 days. It is characterised by becoming tearful at times, irritability and anxiety in situations where one would not normally become anxious. Sleep may also be affected. It usually responds to support and reassurance. Follow-up is important to ensure that the patient has recovered and has not developed a more serious case of PND and a full history should be taken to differentiate between the two. Suicidal tendency is not a feature of baby blues.

8 a

This case sounds more serious than the case in Question 7. Although a clinically useful and acceptable term (to women), there is no evidence that 'PND' is different to depression at any other time in one's life. Symptoms and signs that suggest depression, such as early morning wakening, anhedonia, poor libido, lack of interest, feelings of guilt, poor appetite, weight loss and suicidal ideation should all be sought for in a detailed history when PND is suspected. The NICE questions for depression screening or the Edinburgh Postnatal Depression Scale can be used to screen new mothers for PND.

9 c and e are false

SSRI use is linked with preterm birth and reduced birthweight. A review of 339 cases found that only 11 cases had ECT-related fetal or neonatal complications.

The pregnant mother taking antidepressants is also at an increased risk of developing pre-eclampsia and bleeding.

10   a, c and d

Bipolar disorder is commonly seen in the younger population, making it more likely to be seen in women of childbearing age. Pregnancy has been found to be protective against a recurrence of symptoms of bipolar disorder in some women. Conversely, management is the most difficult when symptoms recur unexpectedly. The risk of recurrence is highest after delivery. Lithium is amongst the most common drugs used for bipolar disorder. However, lithium is commonly associated with an increased risk of Ebstein's anomaly, a rare heart defect in which the tricuspid valve extends into a variably hypoplastic right ventricle. Infants exposed to lithium in utero were found to have an increased birthweight by a mean of 92 g in comparison with non-exposed infants. This was despite the increased incidence of smoking amongst mothers taking lithium. Lithium is secreted in breast milk and can accumulate in the infant due to a lower renal clearance. A specialist with expertise in its use should monitor lithium use in pregnancy and breastfeeding.

11   b

Syphilis is known as the 'great imitator' due to the great variety of its clinical manifestations. It is caused by the spirochaete *Treponema pallidum*. Its clinical manifestations may be divided into primary, secondary, latent (early and late) and tertiary syphilis. This woman has presented with a 'chancre', a painless ulcer associated with primary syphilis. This will usually appear in the first 3 months of infection and may be associated with a non-specific illness. As the ulcer will normally self-resolve, it may be ignored, hence delaying diagnosis. Secondary syphilis is the most contagious phase and may last for 1 to 6 months after the initial infection. The infected patient is most contagious during the primary and secondary stages. Tertiary syphilis will normally occur between 3 and 10 years after the initial infection but may present up to 50 years after the initial infection. Benzathine penicillin is the treatment of choice in primary syphilis. Alternative regimes include azithromycin (2 g orally as a single dose).

12 e

Gonorrhoea is caused by the Gram-negative diplococcus *Neiserria gonorrhoeae*. An altered vaginal discharge may be present in up to 50% of women. Endocervical infection is frequently asymptomatic. Other sites that may get infected include the urethra (causing dysuria), pharynx, rectum and conjunctiva. A combination of ceftriaxone and azithromycin is the current first-line recommended treatment. Patients should avoid sexual intercourse for 7 days after treatment.

13 c

Chlamydia is caused by *Chlamydia trachomatis*. It is a very common STI and may be asymptomatic in 70% of women. Of the regimes listed, azithromycin 1 g given as single oral dose is the most appropriate. Doxycycline at a dose of 100 mg twice per day for 7 days is a suitable alternative regime. If the patient is pregnant or breastfeeding then erythromycin 500 mg four times per day for 7 days (or twice per day for 14 days) may be a more suitable option. Doxycycline is contraindicated in pregnancy. Azithromycin can be used if there is no suitable alternative. Sexual intercourse should be avoided until treatment is completed or until 7 days after treatment if a single dose of azithromycin is used.

14 a, c and d

Neonatal herpes infection is a rare but serious systemic infection associated with high rates of mortality and morbidity. Clinically, it may present in three different forms. In the most common type, lesions are limited to the skin, eyes and mucosa. This accounts for approximately 45% of neonatal infections. Intravenous acyclovir is required and the long-term developmental outcome is good. If treated suboptimally, it has the potential to progress to more severe disease. Cutaneous disease may recur during childhood, requiring recurrent courses of suppressive therapy.

CNS disease accounts for 30% of cases of neonatal HSV. It may present with non-specific symptoms, such as lethargy and poor feeding. Seizures may also be a feature and cutaneous lesions may be present. CNS HSV-2 infection is associated with a greater morbidity. Children with CNS disease have high rates of developmental problems. The highest fatality rate is associated with disseminated disease, which accounts for 25% of clinical manifestations. There is multi-organ involvement. Although intravenous acyclovir therapy reduces the mortality rate, the risk of death remains high at 30%.

15 a, c and e

In the UK, where safe feeding alternatives are available, HIV-positive women are advised not to breastfeed. Pre-antiretroviral therapy data suggest that HIV-positive women who breastfeed increase the risk of mother to child transmission from approximately 14% to 28%. Midwives should have a sufficient understanding of HIV and the risks of mother to child transmission to enable them to include HIV antibody testing early in the pregnancy at routine booking investigations. In the absence of intervention, over 80% of transmissions occur late in the third trimester, during labour and at delivery. However, about 2% of transmissions occur in first and second trimester in the absence of intervention. Option c is true; however, if the mother is on antiretroviral therapy and has an undetectable viral load, the benefit of caesarean section is uncertain. As antibodies cross the placenta, making them unreliable for diagnosis at birth, PCR techniques are used for diagnosis of infection in the newborn child. However, the absence of HIV antibodies at 18 months confirms the child is unaffected.

16 g

ECV is performed at 36 weeks in nulliparous women and at 37 weeks in multiparous women. The aim is to change the presentation from breech to cephalic. The success rate for ECV is about 50%, with approximately 3% reverting back to a breech presentation. Some argue for natural methods of version, such as acupuncture and the assumption of certain postures, but their efficacy is unclear. ECV is a safe procedure but CTG facilities should be nearby, as approximately 0.5% will require immediate delivery by caesarean section due to either abnormalities in the fetal heart rate or vaginal bleeding. ECV can be painful and tocolytics such as salbutamol or terbutaline may be used to improve the chances of a successful ECV. This is a potentially sensitising event, so RhD-negative mothers should receive anti-D Ig.

17 d

The first scan in early pregnancy is ideally carried out at around 12 weeks. This is to determine the number of pregnancies, the gestational age, look for gross congenital anomalies and fetal viability. Crown–rump length can be used before 13 weeks as a method of calculating gestational age. Between 18 and 20 weeks, a more detailed anomaly scan is carried out, which should comment on head shape, spine, abdomen, limbs, renal pelvis and thorax at the level of four-chamber heart view. In some places, facilities may allow comment on cardiac outflow tracts and face and lips to detect cardiac abnormalities and cleft lips. If a low-lying placenta is seen then a further scan should be offered at around 36 weeks to rule out placenta praevia.

18 b

Folic acid is a synthetic form of the B vitamin folate. High folate foods include black-eyed beans, spinach, broccoli, chickpeas and beef and yeast extract. All women should be advised to take 400 µg of folic acid pre-conceptually and for the first 12 weeks of pregnancy. This reduces the risk of spinal cord problems such as spina bifida in the developing fetus. Women who have previously given birth to a child with spinal cord problems should take 5 mg of folic acid daily.

19 d

The dark line running from the xiphisternum to the suprapubic area is known as the 'linea nigra'. It is a type of hyperpigmentation probably due to increased melanin secondary to oestrogen. Other cutaneous signs of pregnancy are striae gravidarum (new stretch marks that have a purplish hue) and striae albicans (silvery-looking old stretch marks). The umbilicus may be everted or flattened due to increased intra-abdominal pressure. An increase in the lumbar lordosis is associated with a normal pregnancy and may lead to lower backache, another common symptom of pregnancy. The uterus becomes palpable at 12 weeks and reaches the umbilicus at about 20 weeks. By 36 weeks, it will have reached the xiphisternum. The SFH measurement is better at identifying small-for-dates, rather than large-for-dates, gestation. At 32 weeks' gestation, the SFH should be 32 ± 2 cm, so 28 cm is too small.

20 e

Options a to d are routinely performed along with a hepatitis B and HIV screen at the booking appointment. A haemoglobinopathy screen may be carried out in individuals deemed at high risk of having abnormal haemoglobin. Routine screening for diabetes is not carried out, partly due to the lack of consensus on when and by what means the diagnosis should be made; it would be reasonable to target individuals at a greater risk of developing diabetes. Fasting plasma glucose, though convenient, will fail to diagnose up to 30% of individuals with diabetes. For this reason, the World Health Organization recommends that the glucose tolerance test be retained as a diagnostic test for diabetes. Carrying the test out later in pregnancy has a higher detection rate but misses the opportunity of early intervention, which would improve pregnancy outcome.

21 b

Open Burch colposuspension is an effective surgical procedure for stress inconti-nence. It involves making a hammock-like structure around the urethra to provide it with support. The procedure is performed via an incision just above the pubic hair line. Alternatively, it can also be done laparoscopically. Open colposuspen-sion achieves continence rates of 85%–90% at 1 year. This falls to 70% at 5 years. Tension-free vaginal tape is another effective procedure and is the most commonly performed procedure for stress incontinence in the UK. It has a cure rate of approximately 94%. It is also simpler than open colposuspension, with lower rates of postoperative complications such as abdominal hernia. Rates of intra-operative complications, such as bladder injury, are higher. Other methods include injection of bulking agents around the bladder and a transobturator tape. Marshall–Marchetti–Krantz colposuspension used to be common but is no longer recommended due to the above mentioned, more effective, procedures.

22 a

'Laparoscopic ovarian electrocautery', or 'ovarian drilling', is a laparoscopic procedure that involves puncturing the ovary with a laser or electrosurgical needle. It has been shown to lower serum androgens and SHBG levels in 60% of subjects. It has also been shown to cause a persistence of ovulation for up to 20 years following the procedure. According to Green-top Guidelines, this procedure should be reserved for selected anovulatory women with a normal BMI or where laparoscopy is indicated for other reasons.

23 f

A history of late miscarriage with preceding spontaneous rupture of membranes and/or painless cervical dilatation suggests the possibility of cervical weakness. The Medical Research Council/ Royal College of Obstetricians and Gynaecologists multicentre trial showed that elective cervical cerclage was associated with a (small) reduction in preterm birth and delivery of very low birthweight babies. This reduction was most marked in women with three or more second-trimester miscarriages or preterm births. However, the use of cervical cerclage was associated with an increased risk of subsequent medical intervention and puerperal pyrexia. Cervical cerclage is carried out transvaginally and involves putting a stitch in the cervix to close it. Transabdominal cerclage has been advocated in women who have had a previously failed transvaginal attempt or with a short and scarred cervix.

24 d

A 'third-degree tear' is defined as injury to the perineum that also involves the anal sphincter complex (either or both external and internal anal sphincter complex). A fourth-degree tear also involves a breach of the rectal mucosa. Due to the extent of the injury, repair should be carried out in theatre under regional or general anaesthesia. Endoanal ultrasound helps in picking up abnormalities in the anatomy of the anal sphincter and should be used in women experiencing pain or incontinence on follow-up after repair. Laxatives, along with antibiotics, prevent wound dehiscence in the post-operative period, therefore should be used according to local protocols.

25 c

Uterine fibroids are amongst the most common tumours of the female reproductive tract. They are benign in nature and more common in Afro-Caribbean women. They may be asymptomatic, in which case there is no need for intervention. Menorrhagia, along with dysmenorrhoea, dyspareunia and urinary symptoms are amongst the most common problems associated with fibroids. Anaemia is commonly found when menorrhagia is problematic. Treatment may include analgesia, hormonal therapies or surgery. Surgical treatments include hysterectomy, myomectomy, endometrial ablation (in selected cases) and uterine fibroid embolisation. The latter involves occluding the vessels around the fibroid with embolising agents, resulting in blockage of blood supply to the fibroid and ischaemic infarction. Most women will experience pain after the procedure. Embolisation is contraindicated in pregnancy or if cancer is suspected. Fibroids tend to shrink in size after the menopause.

26 g

This describes the phenotype for Turner's syndrome, which is the most common sex-chromosome abnormality in females. The diagnosis is confirmed by analysis of the chromosomes (XO). There is ovarian dysgenesis. Secondary sexual characteristics will usually be absent, though sparse growth in the axilla and pubic regions may be stimulated with adrenal androgens, which may sometimes confuse the diagnosis. Newborn infants may be recognised because they are small for dates, have lymphoedema of the hands and feet and excessive skin at the nape of the neck.

27 a

This is suggestive of Asherman's syndrome. This is a syndrome of uterine occlusion secondary to uterine procedures such as curettage or transcervical resection of the endometrium. 'Sheehan's syndrome' is hypopituitarism secondary to post-partum haemorrhage due to pituitary infarction. Perrault syndrome is a rare autosomal recessive disorder resulting in gonadal dysgenesis. It is associated with varying degrees of sensorineural deafness.

28 d

This 16-year-old girl has developed secondary sexual characteristics but has not had a period. The cyclical pain is from her periods but she has an imperforate hymen, which is preventing the flow of blood, hence amenorrhoea is mimicked. This is known as 'haematocolpos', a rare condition. The abdominal mass is the collection of blood in her pelvis. This can be associated with urinary hesitancy and frequency. A bluish membrane, which may be bulging, is seen vaginally in theatre. Treatment is by incising this membrane to release the blood from the uterus. The condition does not have any adverse effect on the ability to conceive.

29 b, c and e

Menorrhagia may be objectively defined as menstrual loss of 80 mL per month. Although studies suggest that only 10% of women may suffer from this level of blood loss, up to a third of women consider their blood loss to be excessive. A FBC is necessary, as it can serve as a surrogate marker of blood loss and help with objective monitoring of the success of treatment. Tranexamic acid may reduce menstrual blood loss by half. NSAIDs such as mefenamic acid may reduce blood loss by a third. Hormonal options include the COCP and the levonorgestrel-releasing intrauterine system (Mirena coil). Cyclical progestogens are also commonly used but are not very effective. Endometrial ablation, which involves destruction of the endometrial lining by laser, electro- or photocoagulation, is a relatively new option. It is a usually well-tolerated and effective option. The most common inherited bleeding disorder responsible for menorrhagia is von Willebrand's disorder. It is caused by a deficiency in von Willebrand factor, which is necessary for normal platelet functioning. Menorrhagia can be associated with ovulatory and non-ovulatory cycles, the latter typically resulting in irregular menstruation.

30 e

Primary ovarian insufficiency is diagnosed when a woman under the age of 40 years presents with amenorrhoea for the preceding 4 months or more and two separate serum FSH levels are in the menopausal range. The second FSH level should be obtained at least 1 month after the first. The diagnosis may also apply if the woman presents with erratic periods with menopausal FSH levels, as ovarian function may be intermittent in the condition also. The underlying cause remains unknown in up to 90% of cases. It may be associated with a number of syndromes, including fragile X-associated disorders. Other potential causes of secondary amenorrhoea include PCOS, hypothalamic amenorrhoea and hyperprolactinaemia. Treatment should include HRT (discussed in detail in Case 11).

31 c

Methyldopa and labetalol are commonly used in pregnancy, along with nifedipine and hydralazine. There have been some concerns regarding β-blockers and the increased risk of IUGR. However, this may only be when the hypertension is treated too aggressively. If β-blockers are used in the third trimester, serial growth scans should be performed to monitor fetal growth. ACE inhibitors, such as ramipril, are contraindicated in pregnancy due to the risk of congenital cardiac and CNS abnormalities.

32 f

Warfarin use between 6 and 12 weeks has been associated with fetal warfarin syndrome, which is manifested as the abnormalities described in this question. Use of warfarin in the latter part of pregnancy has been associated with mental retardation, microcephaly and blindness. If anticoagulation is required in pregnancy, the patient should be switched to unfractionated or low-molecular weight heparin.

33 a

Leflunomide is a relatively new disease-modifying anti-rheumatic drug used in the treatment of rheumatoid arthritis. The mechanism of its action is unclear, though it is thought to interfere with DNA formation. It is contraindicated in pregnancy due to concerns regarding its teratogenicity. Active metabolites of leflunomide have been detected 2 years after the drug has been stopped. Women of childbearing age should be using reliable contraception if taking this drug.

34 a, d and e

CBT, motivational interviewing and support from NHS Stop Smoking Services are all interventions that have been shown to be effective in helping pregnant women to give up smoking. Provision of incentives to help this group stop smoking has been shown to be effective in other countries but research into whether this would be effective in the UK needs to be undertaken (which is unlikely in the current economic climate). There is insufficient data to support Option b. There is mixed evidence regarding the effectiveness of NRT in helping pregnant women stop smoking. However, the NICE guidelines allow for using NRT in pregnancy if it is felt that it would help in the quitting attempt. Varenicline and bupropion should not be offered to pregnant women. Both also lower the seizure threshold so are contraindicated in epilepsy. Cotinine is a breakdown product of nicotine. It has a half-life of approximately 24 hours (as opposed to the 30 minutes of nicotine), allowing exposure to be detected over the previous few days rather than hours (as with CO tests).

35 e

Aplasia cutis is a rare condition in which areas of skin are missing in the newborn. Most commonly the missing areas of skin are on the scalp. Carbimazole has also been associated with choanal and oesophageal atresia. DiGeorge syndrome is typically due to a deletion in chromosome 22 resulting in abnormalities in thymus, parathyroid gland and cardiac development. Dandy–Walker syndrome is a congenital neurological condition in which abnormalities of the cerebellum and the fourth ventricle are present. Warfarin use in the first trimester has been implicated as a cause.

36 c

This woman has pre-eclampsia. The proteinuria needs to be quantified by either a spot urine albumin creatinine ratio or a 24 h protein collection. Proteinuria of >0.3 g in 24 hours with hypertension constitutes pre-eclampsia. Severe hypertension is confirmed by a systolic BP >170 or diastolic BP >110 mmHg on two separate occasions. The RCOG guidelines suggest using a mercury sphygmomanometer for measuring BP, as automated methods may give inaccurate readings. Antihypertensives commonly used include labetalol, nifedipine, methyldopa and hydralazine. Labetalol is contraindicated in this asthmatic woman. ACE inhibitors and angiotensin receptor blockers are contraindicated because of unacceptable adverse effects in the fetus.

37 a

Atosiban is an oxytocin receptor antagonist and has a UK product licence as a tocolytic to prevent preterm labour. Though preterm labour remains the most important cause of adverse infant outcome, it is notoriously difficult to diagnose in the absence of cervical dilatation beyond 3 cm or spontaneous rupture of membranes. In some circumstances, use of tocolytics is justified, for example, when there is the need to give antenatal steroids to prevent fetal respiratory distress syndrome and to organise in utero transfer (as is the case in this question). However, there is insufficient evidence that they have a substantive effect on perinatal or infant mortality, but they are effective in reducing the number of women who deliver within 7 days of commencing the drug. Other tocolytics that may be used are β-agonists such as ritodrine and calcium channel blockers such as nifedipine.

38 j

Cord prolapse is when the umbilical cord protrudes below the presenting part after the rupture of membranes. This can be extremely dangerous, as the umbilical vessels in the cord can be compressed either by direct pressure from the presenting part or from spasm, due to exposure, in the cord. This compromises blood supply to the fetus, hence immediate delivery is required. Management is focused on delivering the fetus as soon as possible and keeping pressure off the presenting part of the cord. Standing the mother upright would be more likely to result in pressure on the cord from the presenting part, so should be avoided. The mother should be asked to assume the knee-to-chest position. Handling the cord increases the risk of spasm. Saline in the bladder can help in displacing the presenting part upwards.

39 d

There are four categories of caesarean section, as determined by the urgency with which the procedure is required. Category 1 should be carried out within 30 minutes, as there is an immediate threat to either the mother or the child (this is commonly known as a 'crash C section' on the ward). Category 2 refers to an urgent section when there is a non-immediate threat to either life. Category 3 is a scheduled caesarean section where there is no fetomaternal compromise but early delivery is required. Primary genital herpes in the third trimester is an indication for category 4, or 'elective C section', in which delivery is timed to suit the patient and staff.

40 b

Neonatal resuscitation follows the same principle of 'airway, breathing, circulation' used in other resuscitations. The first step in routine neonatal care is to provide warmth and stimulation by rubbing the newborn dry, wrapping in dry towels and placing under a heater if available. This allows for monitoring of vital signs. Due to the large occiput, the head should be placed in a neutral position, in which it is neither extended nor flexed. If the baby is not breathing by 90 seconds, then five inflation breaths must be given. Since, by now, the lungs are filled with fluid, these breaths need to be of 2–3 seconds duration and of a sustained pressure of about 30 cm of water. If the heart rate is not already at or above 100 bpm, in most cases this will lift it to this rate. Chest compressions start if the heart rate does not recover above 60 bpm.

41 i

42 b

43 e

No form of immunisation can be considered completely safe in pregnancy due to the lack of studies in this area. In each case, the potential risks of contracting illness need to be weighed against the benefits (and potential risks) of giving the vaccine, toxoid or Ig. The benefit of vaccination is likely to be greater when the risk of contracting the disease is high. Live vaccines such as measles, mumps and rubella (MMR), yellow fever, varicella and oral polio vaccine (Sabin) should be avoided in pregnancy. Cholera vaccine is no longer recommended for international travel, as it is not considered very effective. Travellers should be encouraged to pay special attention to personal and food and water hygiene to prevent contracting the illness. Neonatal tetanus is a serious condition that accounted for approximately 130 000 deaths globally in 2004. Two doses of tetanus toxoid, 4 weeks apart, in pregnant women or women of childbearing age, has a significant impact on reducing the risk of neonatal tetanus.

44 c

45 d

Antiretroviral therapy to mother and neonate, elective caesarean section and avoidance of breastfeeding are all interventions shown to reduce the risk of verti- cal transmission. A combination of these three interventions is associated with a vertical transmission rate of <2%. If the mother is on antiretroviral therapy and has an undetectable viral load, the benefit of caesarean section is uncertain. Some women will prefer to avoid caesarean section and this should be an important consideration in the final decision regarding mode of delivery. If a planned vagi- nal delivery is chosen, then the membranes should be left intact for as long as possible. Use of fetal scalp electrodes and fetal blood sampling should also be avoided. The cord should be clamped as early as possible after delivery and the baby should be bathed immediately after birth.

46 a

In the UK, 15% of women are RhD negative. The chance of the baby being RhD positive depends on whether the father is homozygous DD (100% chance) or het- erozygous Dd (50% chance). 'Non-sensitised' refers to the fact that this woman has not been exposed to RhD-positive blood, hence does not have antibodies. The RCOG guidelines state the risk of sensitisation by spontaneous miscarriage before 12 weeks' gestation is negligible when there has been no instrumentation to evacuate the products of conception and, therefore, anti-D Ig is not required in these circumstances.

47 f

This question refers to the routine care of non-sensitised RhD-negative women in pregnancy, which is discussed in Answer 46. The other option is a single higher dose at 28 weeks.

48 d

49 a, b and d

SCD consists of a number of single-gene autosomal recessive disorders characterised by the presence of the 'sickle' gene (S). The presence of the sickle gene impacts the structure of haemoglobin (Hb), which polymerises in low oxygen conditions. This polymerisation leads to the increased breakdown of cells (anaemia) and sequestration of cells in the small blood vessels (painful crisis, stroke, pulmonary embolism, renal impairment). Two copies of the sickle gene are present in sickle cell anaemia (HbSS) and single copies when it is coupled with other abnormal haemoglobins, Hb C and beta thalassaemia amongst others. Each genotype is associated with disease of varying severity. Primary care physicians should encourage partner haemoglobinopathy screening and refer for pre-implantation genetic diagnosis if appropriate. This involves performing in vitro fertilisation followed by removal of cells from the resulting blastomeres on day 3. PCR is then used to look for haemoglobinopathy mutations within the cells removed. The normal blastomeres are identified and selected for implantation. In the event of a painful crisis, the World Health Organization pain ladder should be used. Pethidine is associated with an increased risk of seizures in SCD and should be avoided. SCD in itself is not an indication for caesarean section, which should only be carried out if there are other obstetric indications for doing so. Birth should be undertaken in hospital between 38 and 40 weeks to minimise the risk of complications associated with a later delivery.

50 c

As SCD sufferers are in a hyposplenic state, they are at risk of infection by encapsulated organisms. Despite a lack of clear data, the RCOG recommends prophylaxis with penicillin. In the presence of an allergy to penicillin, erythromycin should be used. If not already covered, women should be offered *Haemophilus influenzae* type B and conjugated meningococcal C (combined), pneumococcal, hepatitis B, swine flu and influenza vaccines. The higher dose of folic acid is recommended. SCD is considered a mild risk factor for the development of pre-eclampsia, so aspirin may be considered in this patient. Hydroxycarbamide is used to reduce the incidence of painful crises but is teratogenic in animals. It is therefore recommended that it be stopped 3 months prior to conception. In cases where inadvertent exposure has taken place, no adverse effects to the fetus have been reported. ACE inhibitors such as ramipril are commonly used in the outlined scenario. However, second- and third-trimester exposure has been associated with oligohydramnios, renal failure, anuria and fetal death and first-trimester use is associated with cardiovascular and CNS malformations. Therefore, the ramipril should be stopped.

51 e

CTPA is considered the investigative modality of choice for the diagnosis of non-massive pulmonary embolus. In comparison with perfusion lung scans, it is associated with a lower fetal radiation exposure (0.01 mGy). The risk of fetal cancer with the former is estimated at 1 in 280 000. However, CTPA is associated with a greater radiation dose to the female breast (10 mGy compared with 0.28 mGy with a perfusion scan). This confers a small increase in the risk of breast cancer in the woman.

52 f

Various screening tests are available for Down's syndrome. The risk of Down's syndrome increases with increasing maternal age. An important study that looked into the safety and cost-effectiveness of screening for Down's syndrome was the Serum Urine and Ultrasound Screening Study. The study concluded that the integrated test is the safest and most effective method. This test involves a nuchal USS (at 10–13 + 6 weeks) and a blood test measuring pregnancy-associated plasma protein A at 10 weeks. This is followed by a quadruple test measuring oestriol, hCG, α-fetoprotein and inhibin A at 15 weeks. It has a detection rate of 85% with a false positive rate of 1.2%.

53 d

This is the generally accepted figure for rate of miscarriage associated with amniocentesis. Amniocentesis is normally performed between 15 and 20 weeks. If earlier diagnosis is required, chorionic villus sampling may be performed between 10 and 13 weeks. Early amniocentesis (prior to 14 completed weeks) is associated with a higher rate of fetal loss, an increased incidence of fetal talipes and respiratory morbidity compared with other procedures.

54 b

The harms of smoking in pregnancy are well established. It is associated with miscarriage, placental abruption, premature birth (rather than delayed onset) and ectopic pregnancy. Babies born to smoking mothers are on average 200 g smaller than those born to comparable non-smoking mothers. Congenital defects and stillbirths are also more common. There is also evidence that children born to smoking mothers have lower achievements in reading and maths. A recent study in the *British Journal of Obstetrics and Gynaecology* has shown that smoking is related to an increased incidence of pelvic pain. In this nested case-control study, 2302 smokers were compared with 2692 non-smokers; a significant increase in the incidence of pelvic pain was noted in the former. Vasoconstriction and local ischemia may be the responsible underlying pathophysiology.

55 c

Plasmin is formed from the activation of plasminogen. It is a key player in the fibrinolytic pathway, attacking fibrin (the major component of a clot) at 50 different sites, thereby reducing its size. Antithrombin III is a plasmin inhibitor. The oral contraceptive pill also reduces the activity of plasmin. Reduction in plasmin activity renders a pro-thrombotic state. Deficiency in protein C, also a major component of the coagulation system, increases the risks of clots. Trousseau's syndrome describes the increased risk of coagulopathy in the presence of cancer. Antiphospholipid syndrome is associated with an increased risk of VTE and pregnancy losses. The presence of antiphospholipid antibodies has also been associated with premature delivery. Factor VIII deficiency or absence is the underlying problem in haemophilia A, which increases the risk of bleeding.

56   d

Sex-cord stromal tumours account for about 5% of ovarian tumours. Sertoli–Leydig cell tumours are a rare type of sex-cord stromal tumours. Patients may present with signs of virilisation due to excessive testosterone production by the tumour. The tumour is usually benign and unilateral. Management is determined by the age of presentation and stage and differentiation of the tumour.

57   e

Meigs' syndrome is a rare disease complex consisting of a benign ovarian tumour (classically, a fibroma), ascites and pleural effusion. The mechanism by which fluid collects in the peritoneal cavity and pleural space is unclear. However, removal of the tumour results in resolution of the fluid. Ascites and pleural effusion may also occur with ovarian malignancies.

58   a

Ovarian torsion occurs when the ovarian pedicle rotates on its long axis, cutting off venous and lymphatic drainage. Prolonged torsion can cause venous and arterial thrombosis resulting in ovarian infarction. Pregnancy (due to laxity of supporting tissues) and ovulation induction (possibly due to enlarged ovaries as a result of multiple maturing follicles) increase the risk of torsion. The list of differential diagnoses is long, making diagnosis difficult, as any cause of an acute abdomen may mimic ovarian torsion. White cell count may be raised. Treatment may involve untwisting of the adnexa or surgical removal of the ovary.

59 d

The FIGO scoring system is used to stage gynaecological cancers. Wells' score and modified Wells' score are used in the diagnosis of DVT and pulmonary embolus, respectively. The RMI 1 and 2 are used to determine the risk of malignancy in a pelvic mass. Scores based on ultrasound features, the woman's menopausal state and Ca-125 levels are used to determine the final score. The MASI is used to determine the severity of melasma. The nine most androgen-sensitive areas of the body are given a score of 1 to 4, depending on the severity of hairiness. This is then used to calculate the Ferriman–Gallwey score. A score >8 suggests hirsutism. The scoring system is subjective and does not take into account the degree to which the problem affects the patient's quality of life.

60 b and c

Bilateral ovarian wedge resection was the first surgical treatment used to induce ovulation in women with PCOS. The introduction of agents such as clomiphene resulted in the temporary abandonment of surgical methods. Laparoscopy revived the use of surgical methods and currently the most widely used technique is laparoscopic ovarian diathermy using electrocautery. Approximately four in five women will ovulate after LOS, if they fail to respond to clomiphene, and half will fall pregnant. Although LOS does reduce levels of circulating androgens, its role in the treatment of acne and hirsutism has not been studied. LOS, however, does not improve insulin resistance or the mentioned lipoprotein abnormalities. Older surgical techniques have been associated with an increased risk of developing hypertension and diabetes later in life.

61 b

Deficiency in the B vitamins (particularly folate, riboflavin, B6 and B12) is associated with homocysteinemia. Elevated plasma homocysteine concentrations have been associated with adverse pregnancy outcomes such as placental abruptions, stillbirths, preterm birth and low birthweight. Although homocysteine levels drop in pregnancy anyway, supplementation with folic acid in the latter two trimesters has been associated with an enhanced reduction in levels. Elevated homocysteine levels have also been linked to high coffee intake and cigarette smoking. However, due to the lack of strong evidence to support their benefit, supplementation is not routinely recommended with any of the B vitamins (except folic acid).

62   a

High doses of vitamin A early in pregnancy are potentially teratogenic. RCOG recommends an intake of no more than 700 mcg/day (approximately 2300 IU/day). Doses of 3000 mcg/day (10 000 IU/day) or more have been associated with birth defects. One study estimated that amongst women who took more than 10 000 IU/day, 1 in every 57 babies born with a birth defect was due to high maternal intake of vitamin A. Liver and liver products are high in vitamin A. Women should be advised to avoid excessive consumption in pregnancy.

63   f

Copper serves as an important cofactor to a number of enzymes. Levels of copper increase during pregnancy, possibly due to altered ceruloplasmin synthesis, which is the major copper-binding protein in blood. Low levels of ceruloplasmin are associated with Wilson's disease, an inherited disorder of excess copper. A maternal diet low in copper has been associated with embryonic death and gross structural abnormalities.

64   e

Periconceptual folic acid, up to 12 weeks' gestation, is recommended at a dose of 400 mcg/day. This is associated with a reduced risk of neural tube, congenital heart and limb defects. It also seems to protect against the risk of some paediatric cancers such as leukaemia, brain tumours and neuroblastomas. There have been some concerns regarding an increased rate of twin births associated with folic acid supplementation in pregnancy.

65   a and b

Zinc deficiency has been associated with prolonged labour, pre-eclampsia, fetal growth restriction and death. Zinc supplementation in pregnancy has been associated with greater birthweight and head circumference. Smoking appears to increase the metabolic turnover of vitamin C, thereby increasing the requirements of smokers. High-dose vitamin C supplementation is not recommended. Vitamin D supplementation in pregnancy is associated with a reduced risk of type 1 diabetes in childhood. The Healthy Start multivitamin tablet, recommended for pregnancy by the NHS, contains 70 mg of vitamin C, 10 mcg of vitamin D and 400 mcg of folic acid.

66   h

67   i

68   c

'Paraphilia' refers to a group of psychosexual disorders characterised by sexual fantasies, urges or gratification through non-human objects or situations, children or non-consenting partners. To be diagnosed as a disorder, the behaviour has to cause marked distress or interpersonal difficulty. Fantasies and urges, strong enough to cause distress, are sufficient for the diagnosis and the actual carrying out of the behaviour is not necessary. Symptoms should be present over a period of 6 months. Since the woman in Question 67 is not distressed, she does not fulfil the diagnostic criteria for exhibitionistic disorder, where sexual pleasure is derived from the exposure of one's genitals to unsuspecting strangers. Fetishistic disorder involves deriving pleasure from the use of inanimate objects in a sexual manner (e.g. female undergarments). In sexual masochism, pleasure is derived from one's own suffering, whereas, in sexual sadism, pleasure is derived from the suffering of another person. Transvestic disorder applies only to heterosexual males (though this aspect of the definition may be dropped in the fifth edition of the *Diagnostic and Statistical Manual of Mental Disorders*, due in 2013) where sexual pleasure is derived from cross-dressing.

69   b and c

There is a lack of consensus on the definition of 'vaginismus'. However, it generally refers to the difficulty associated with allowing vaginal entry to any object, despite the desire to allow it. Other definitions refer to it as involuntary spasm of the outer third of the vagina, resulting in interference with intercourse. The patient may continue to experience sexual pleasure through alternative stimulation. Primary vaginismus is lifelong and is a common cause of non-consummation of marriage. This patient is suffering from secondary vaginismus, as it has occurred after sexual function has been normal (not because she allows the entry of certain objects) as is evident from the birth of their child. A physically traumatic childbirth may result in secondary vaginismus. Other organic conditions that may lead to vaginismus include atrophic vaginitis, vulvovaginitis, vulvar dermatoses and endometriosis. The lack of good quality studies means that it is difficult to ascertain the underlying aetiology of vaginismus. Themes that recur in the literature include negative views regarding sex in general, fear of sex, belief that sex is wrong or shameful, traumatic early childhood experiences and sexual abuse.

70   All of the options

Various techniques have been used to manage vaginismus. The evidence for their use is not well established. Desensitisation involves exposure to situations that would normally provoke fear and anxiety in a graded manner. In the context of vaginismus, this involves the introduction of vaginal trainers, gradually increasing in size until one can admit a trainer similar in size to their partner's penis. Progressive relaxation is a means of relaxing muscles. This may allow vaginal entry if pelvic floor muscles are relaxed. Sensate focus, which has been discussed in this case of FSD, involves a gradual progress in intimacy from touch to penetration. Electromyography may be used to detect pelvic floor muscle contraction. This allows the patient to become aware of unintentional muscle spasm. They may then use relaxation techniques to allow intercourse to occur. CBT has also been shown to be beneficial. Other treatments for which reports exist include topical lidocaine applied in the vagina, botulinum toxin injected into the puborectalis muscles and intravenous diazepam.

71 b

Obstetric cholestasis, also referred to as 'intrahepatic cholestasis of pregnancy', is a condition of pregnancy in which there is pruritus in the absence of a rash with deranged LFTs. Pruritus affects the palms and soles in particular. It will normally occur in the latter half of pregnancy and resolve after delivery. The risk of harm to the mother is low. However, it is associated with an increased risk of preterm birth and fetal death. A raised serum bile-acid concentration is important for the diagnosis. Ursodeoxycholic acid can help reduce plasma bile-acid concentration and pruritus.

72 i

This case is suggestive of primary biliary cirrhosis (PBC). PBC is an autoimmune disease leading to slow but progressive destruction of the intrahepatic bile ducts and possible cirrhosis. It mainly affects women and is more common in the fifth decade of life. Although the majority of patients are diagnosed when asymptomatic, approximately one in five patients will present with non-specific malaise and pruritus. Of patients with PBC, 5%–10% will have no detectable AMAs. Ursodeoxycholic acid can be used safely in pregnancy. Liver transplantation has improved survival rates in patients with PBC.

73 e

HELLP syndrome is characterised by haemolysis, elevated liver enzymes and low platelets. The abnormalities seen on blood testing are suggested by the name. A raised BP and proteinuria may be present in 85% of cases, suggesting an overlap with pre-eclampsia. Approximately 10% of women with pre-eclampsia will develop HELLP. Management is focused on expediting delivery, as liver damage can be accelerated, with potential fatal consequences for the mother and child. Acute fatty liver of pregnancy, a rare but serious condition, should be considered as an alternative diagnosis.

74   a, c and d

Oedema is not necessarily required to diagnose pre-eclampsia, though it may often be present. Pre-eclampsia is characterised by hypertension and proteinuria of 300 mg or more over 24 hours. It is diagnosed after the 20th gestational week. Symptoms occurring within 48 hours of delivery would also meet the diagnostic criteria. The onset of seizures heralds eclampsia. Budd–Chiari syndrome involves an obstruction of the hepatic veins. Doppler ultrasound is used to aid diagnosis. The Swansea diagnostic criteria are used for the diagnosis of acute fatty liver of pregnancy.

75   a

Vertical transmission is the most common mode of HBV transmission in endemic areas. HBV viral load plays a crucial role in the risk of vertical transmission. If the viral load is high, the risk of transmission may be as high as 90%. Transmission may also occur through breastfeeding. The mode of delivery, vaginal or cae-sarean, does not affect the risk of transmission. Giving the infant hepatitis B Ig within 12 hours of birth can reduce the risk of transmission. Three doses of HBV vaccine should then be administered in the first 6 months of life. The use of antiviral treatment in the final trimester to reduce the risk of transmission is controversial due to concerns regarding viral resistance. Though the risk of vertical transmission of HCV is low, it is increased if the mother also suffers from HIV.

76   e

This question requires knowledge of the UK medical eligibility criteria (UKMEC) for contraceptive use. These criteria advise on the use of contraceptives in the presence of other medical situations. There are four categories:

UKMEC 1: unrestricted use allowed

UKMEC 2: benefits generally outweigh harm

UKMEC 3: risks generally outweigh benefits

UKMEC 4: use represents unacceptable health risk.

The COCP is absolutely contraindicated in those with a personal history of VTE. The POP carries a UKMEC 2 recommendation.

77 j

Emergency contraception is used to prevent an unwanted pregnancy as a result of either UPSI or contraceptive failure. It can be delivered by one of two methods: oral emergency contraception, such as Levonelle 1500, or copper intrauterine contraceptive device. The oral method is 1.5 mg of the progesterone levonorgestrel. It is licensed for use up to 72 hours after UPSI but can be used up to 120 hours after the episode. Efficacy is poor after 72 hours. In this case, 6 days have elapsed, so the copper coil is a more suitable option. It too should be inserted within 120 hours but can be used if the date of ovulation can be reliably predicted and 5 days have not elapsed since the possible date of ovulation (as is the probable case in this scenario). If more than this time has elapsed, proceedings for termination of pregnancy should be initiated (if pregnancy is confirmed and the patient wishes to go ahead).

78 d

In this scenario, the patient requires protection from STIs along with contraception to prevent pregnancy. In young sexually active women, opportunistic health promotion should always be undertaken. She has been fortunate not to have fallen pregnant so far. Condoms are highly effective in preventing STIs and she should be encouraged to ask her partner to use one. She should also use a female condom. With her history, she would be a good candidate for either the OCP or POP. LARCs are probably not an option here due to her needle phobia. Never having had children, she would probably not be keen on intrauterine contraceptive devices. They also increase the risk of infection, making them inappropriate for her at the moment.

79 b

Dianette is a COC containing ethinyloestradiol and cyprotenone acetate. The latter is a progestogen with anti-androgenic properties. It has a licence for the treatment of acne and hirsutism but not as a contraceptive. Due to the increased risk of VTE associated with Dianette, the Committee on the Safety of Medicines advises that it be used as an option for treatment of severe resistant acne or severe hirsutism and be withdrawn 3–4 months after the condition has resolved. UKMEC advises on the safety of contraceptives and knowledge of this is useful for appropriate prescribing. A first-degree relative under the age of 45 years with a history of VTE is a UKMEC 3 for COC use; that is, the risks outweigh the benefits. If the first-degree relative is over the age of 45 years, then it is a UKMEC 2 – the benefits outweigh the risks. The POP is a UKMEC 1, thus unrestricted use is allowed.

80 b

Tubal occlusion may be carried out at any time in the cycle provided the surgeon is confident the patient is not pregnant. Otherwise, the procedure should be carried out in the follicular phase of the cycle preceded by effective contraceptive use or abstinence. Consent should be obtained in advance. The patient should be made aware that sterilisation carried out post-partum is associated with greater regret and a higher failure rate. The procedure can be performed laparoscopically or by mini laparotomy. Filshie® clips or rings are the preferred means of tubal occlusion when performed laparoscopically. Diathermy is harder to reverse and associated with an increased risk of ectopic pregnancy in subsequent pregnancies. Sterilisation may be performed under local anaesthesia. A modified Pomeroy procedure is commonly used at the time of caesarean section. A recent systematic review has found no differences in the complication rates between Filshie® clips and the modified Pomeroy method when performed in the post-partum period. However, the Filshie® clip procedure has been reported to be easier to perform.

81 f

Lichen planus is an inflammatory condition of unknown cause that may affect the skin, oral cavity, genitalia, hair and nails. On the skin, it will typically present as itchy, polygonal, flat-topped papules. The reticulated white streaks are known as Wickham's striae. A punch biopsy of the rash will reveal the described histology. Steroids form the mainstay of treatment.

82 d

Trichomoniasis is a STI caused by the intracellular parasite *Trichomonas vaginalis*. It is more common in women who have more than one sexual partner and who have sex twice or more per week. Mobile trichomonads are seen on a wet mount. Treatment is with oral metronidazole or tinidazole.

83 i

Atrophic vaginitis is caused by a lack of oestrogen. A mild discharge may be associated with the condition. Therefore, infective causes of vulvovaginitis should be ruled out. It may also be associated with urinary symptoms such as dysuria and urinary incontinence. Treatment is usually with topical HRT.

84 b and d

HPV types 6 and 11 are implicated in genital warts, whereas types 16 and 18 cause the majority of cervical cancer cases. Two vaccines are licensed for use against HPV: Cervarix®, which is active against HPV types 16 and 18, and Gardasil®, the quadrivalent vaccine against types 6, 11, 16 and 18. The Department of Health opted for Cervarix®, which is now part of the routine immunisation schedule in the UK and offered to girls between the ages of 12 and 13 years. Podophyllotoxin and imiquimod are effective against genital warts and allow safe treatment at home.

85 a and b

There is no evidence that prophylactic topical acyclovir reduces the risk of acquiring herpes infection. Similarly, avoiding penetrative sex in the absence of condoms may still transmit the virus, as skin-to-skin contact may be sufficient to pass on the virus. It may be advisable to abstain from sex in the third trimester, as acquisition in this trimester is associated with the highest risk to the neonate.

86 a

Hereditary non-polyposis colorectal cancer, also known as 'Lynch syndrome', is associated with an increased risk of developing colorectal, endometrial, ovarian, stomach and hepatobiliary cancers. It is inherited in an autosomal dominant pattern and there is a 40%–60% lifetime risk of developing endometrial carcinoma. Endometrial carcinoma normally presents with postmenopausal bleeding. However, in younger women, it may present with menstrual disturbance.

87 h

Lichen sclerosus is a chronic inflammatory skin condition that may occur anywhere but is particularly common in the anogenital area. It is more common in adult women and can be a source of great distress as it may cause itchiness and dyspareunia. Anogenital lichen sclerosus requires long-term follow-up due to an approximately 5% lifetime risk of developing vulval squamous cell carcinoma. Any suspicious lesions should be biopsied. Topical steroids form the mainstay of treatment for lichen sclerosus. Other agents that have been used include topical testosterone, topical progesterone and retinoids.

88 c

Primary vaginal carcinomas are rare in all ages but are particularly rare in younger women. Squamous cell carcinomas are the most common primary vaginal tumours affecting elderly women. Between 1940 and 1971, diethylstilbestrol, the first synthetic oestrogen developed, was used to prevent complications of pregnancy. Though its popularity declined due to ineffectiveness, complications associated with its use began to emerge later. It is strongly associated with the risk of developing adenocarcinoma of the vagina and cervix in in utero exposed women. These women are also at increased risk of infertility and ectopic pregnancies. They may also be at an increased risk of developing breast cancer after the age of 40 years.

89 a and e are true

GTD encompasses a number of pregnancy-related conditions arising from abnormal trophoblastic cells of the placenta. These include:

- partial hydatidiform mole
- complete hydatidiform mole
- invasive mole

- choriocarcinoma
- placental-site trophoblastic tumour.

The first two are pre-malignant conditions. The latter three are collectively termed 'GTNs' and are malignant conditions. Measurement of hCG forms the basis of diagnosis and management of GTD (rather than Ca-125), as its levels correlate well with the severity of disease. Although the majority of cases of complete hydatidiform moles occur randomly, a rare familial syndrome causing recurrent disease has been identified. These families are aiding research into the condition with the hope of finding an underlying genetic basis. Choriocarcinoma is much more rare than the above-quoted figure of 1 in 1000 and is considered to have an incidence of 1 in 50000 following a non-molar pregnancy.

90 c

Breslow thickness is a measure of the depth of a melanoma, as this is directly related to the prognosis. Ultrasonography is used in the diagnosis of GTN. A vascular mass in the absence of a fetus with a raised hCG suggests GTN. Calculation of the pusatility index allows determination of the degree of arteriovenous shunting across the mass. Due to increased arteriovenous shunting, molar tissue has a low resistance. A low pulsatility index, measured by Doppler studies, is a poor prognostic factor. A chest X-ray will look for lung metastases. If present, this may indicate CNS disease. Hence, lumbar puncture is performed to measure the hCG levels in cerebrospinal fluid. Imaging of the brain, pelvis and abdomen would complete the staging process.

91 g

This scenario of raised BP with proteinuria suggests the possibility of a serious obstetric complication called 'HELLP syndrome'. This can be regarded as a variant of severe pre-eclampsia. It manifests as haemolysis (H), elevated LFTs (EL) and low platelet count (LP). It is a potentially fatal complication, with maternal mortality around 1% and a much higher fetal mortality. Other investigations indicated in

HELLP syndrome are clotting (due to risk of disseminated intravascular coagulation) and a liver ultrasound. The priority in management is to safely deliver a healthy baby. Treatment is otherwise supportive and is the same as in eclampsia; that is, bringing BP down, preventing convulsions, minimising organ damage and controlling coagulopathy.

92 f

This scenario suggests possible urinary bacteraemia. The shaking episode described is typical of rigors that suggest infection. Of the list of investigations available, urinalysis is the one most likely to identify the source of infection. The combination of a tachycardia with a low BP suggests sepsis. Antibiotics and intravenous fluid support are crucial to the care of this patient.

93 b

In a pregnant woman who is itching with no obvious rash, obstetric cholestasis needs ruling out. This affects 0.7% of pregnancies in the UK. It is more common in Asians. Risks for the fetus include preterm labour and, more worryingly, stillbirth. In obstetric cholestasis, LFTs are abnormal and bile acids are raised. Since it is a diagnosis of exclusion, other tests will also need to be performed if LFTs are found to be normal. These may include a clotting screen, USS of the liver biliary system, viral serology for hepatitis, *Cytomegalovirus* and Epstein–Barr virus, and autoimmune screen to rule out conditions such as PBC and chronic active hepatitis. One must be aware that itching can start before LFTs become abnormal. LFTs should, therefore, be repeated if the symptoms persist. There is very little of proven benefit that can be used in cholestasis; however, emollients, antihistamines and ursodeoxycholic acid are commonly used on obstetric units.

94 c

Graves' disease accounts for about 95% of thyrotoxicosis. It presents as weight loss; anxiety; sweatiness; tremor; tachycardia, with or without palpitations; and eye signs. The underlying pathophysiology is the production of TSH-receptor-stimulating antibodies, which causes high free T4 and T3 with subsequent low

TSH. Untreated, it can cause sub-fertility, increase risk of miscarriage, premature delivery and fetal growth restriction. Carbimazole and propylthiouracil are the two drugs used to treat thyrotoxicosis. However, they do cross the placenta and can cause fetal hypothyroidism in high doses. Thyroidectomy is also a viable option in pregnancy. Monitoring is by measuring TSH, T3 and T4 values, which vary in each trimester.

95   a and b

Chronic hypertension during pregnancy is associated with an increased risk of adverse outcomes. This includes an increased risk of pre-eclampsia, fetal growth restriction, preterm birth and placental abruption. In normotensive patients, BP drops towards the end of the first trimester. The same also occurs in the majority of hypertensive women. BP then returns to pre-pregnancy levels towards the end of the third trimester. However, up to a fifth of women may experience a worsening in their BP during pregnancy. The risk of developing pre-eclampsia is approximately 20%. ACE inhibitors should be avoided in pregnancy, as their use has been associated with a number of adverse outcomes for the fetus. Methyldopa, β-blockers such as labetalol and long-acting calcium channel blockers such as nifedipine are considered safe in pregnancy.

96   b

This scenario looks at the primary prevention of osteoporosis. There are concerns regarding osteoporosis in this patient, but we do not have confirmation from a DEXA scan. Since this patient is unwilling to travel, a clinical decision needs to be made. The NICE guidance states that a diagnosis of osteoporosis can be assumed in women aged 75 years and over if obtaining a DEXA scan is clinically inappropriate or unfeasible. However, to initiate treatment for primary prevention, the patient must also have two or more independent clinical risk factors for fracture (family history, alcohol intake greater than four units a week, rheumatoid arthritis) or indicators of low BMD (BMI <21 kg/m^2, certain inflammatory conditions, prolonged immobility, untreated menopause). Since this 80-year-old fulfils this criteria, first-line treatment, which is alendronate, may be initiated.

97 c

This case looks at secondary prevention of osteoporosis, as the patient has already sustained a fracture. She has no independent clinical risk factors for fracture. Since her BMD is below –3.0 she would qualify for treatment with risedronate. Another option would be etidronate (not listed). If she were unable to tolerate either of the two, we would be faced with another 'unresolvable' situation with regard to the NICE guidance. Strontium ranelate and raloxifene, which would be considered next, are only recommended when the T-score drops to –4.0 or below in this age group.

98 e

The NICE guidance recommends teriparatide for the secondary prevention of osteoporosis if the mentioned drugs are not tolerated or the patient suffers another fragility fracture despite adhering to treatment for at least 1 year and there is a drop in the BMD. In the presence of only two fractures, the patient has to be above the age of 65 years with a T-score of –4.0 or below. Younger patients have to have a combination of T-scores below –4.0 and more than two fractures.

99 a

Stress incontinence is the most common urinary complaint in women, affecting up to 10% of women at some point in their life. Leakage of urine is present in up to 40% of postmenopausal women. Duloxetine is the only treatment that is licensed for use in the management of 'urinary stress incontinence', which is defined as the involuntary loss of urine when an increase in abdominal pressure (as a result of coughing, sneezing, laughing, etc.) results in bladder pressure overcoming urethral resistance. Surgical techniques used to manage the condition are discussed in Answer 21 on p. 146. Oxybutynin is an antimuscuranic drug used in the management of OAB. Doxazosin is an α-blocker used in benign prostatic hyperplasia. Like duloxetine, imipramine is also an antidepressant, but it is used in OAB due to its antimuscuranic effects. Duloxetine, a SNRI, can be started at a dose of 20 mg twice daily and gradually increased to 40 mg twice daily. The evidence for the benefit of the α-agonist clonidine in the management of stress incontinence is unconvincing. Important conservative measures include losing weight, cessation of smoking, cutting down caffeine intake, pelvic floor exercises (30–50 daily contractions) and the use of absorptive pads.

100   a, c and e

OAB is a common and troublesome condition associated with urgency and frequency with or without incontinence. The underlying problem is thought to be detrusor overactivity. Detrusor overactivity is an urodynamic observation (hence, not diagnosable from history) where involuntary contractions of the detrusor muscle of the bladder are seen. These contractions may be spontaneous or pro- voked by actions such as coughing or sneezing. When provoked, it may become clinically difficult to distinguish between OAB and stress incontinence. Often these conditions are present concomitantly. A diagnosis of OAB may be made from a good history. Most cases of OAB are idiopathic; however, occasionally it may be due to neurological conditions such as spina bifida, pelvic surgery or mechanical outflow obstruction (more common in men). Antimuscuranics work by relaxing the detrusor muscle. They are associated with troublesome side effects such as dry mouth, constipation, dizziness and blurred vision. The likelihood of side effects may be reduced by gradually increasing the dose or use of sustained-release preparations. Alternative routes of administration, such as a transdermal patch, may also be considered. Botulinum toxin injections into the detrusor muscle under local anaesthetic are being used more commonly to delay the need for surgery, the latter having a poor rate of efficacy and high rate of complications. Botulinum toxin appears to offer good short-term relief. Injections need to be repeated every 6–12 months. However, this treatment does carry the risk of urinary retention, with up to a quarter of patients requiring intermittent self-catheterisation. Other options include desmopressin, topical oestrogen and antidepressants such as imipramine.

Index

Please note: page numbers in brackets ( ) refer to exam practice 'answers'.

DATE DUE
